Sleep Well, Dream Well

Sleep Well, Dream Well

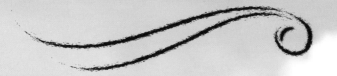

MY NIGHT-TIME JOURNAL

FELICITY FORSTER

ARCTURUS

Picture credit:

All images from Shutterstock

For Tim

ARCTURUS

This edition published in 2020 by Arcturus Publishing Limited
26/27 Bickels Yard, 151–153 Bermondsey Street,
London SE1 3HA

ISBN: 978-1-78950-797-3
AD007506UK

Printed in China

Contents

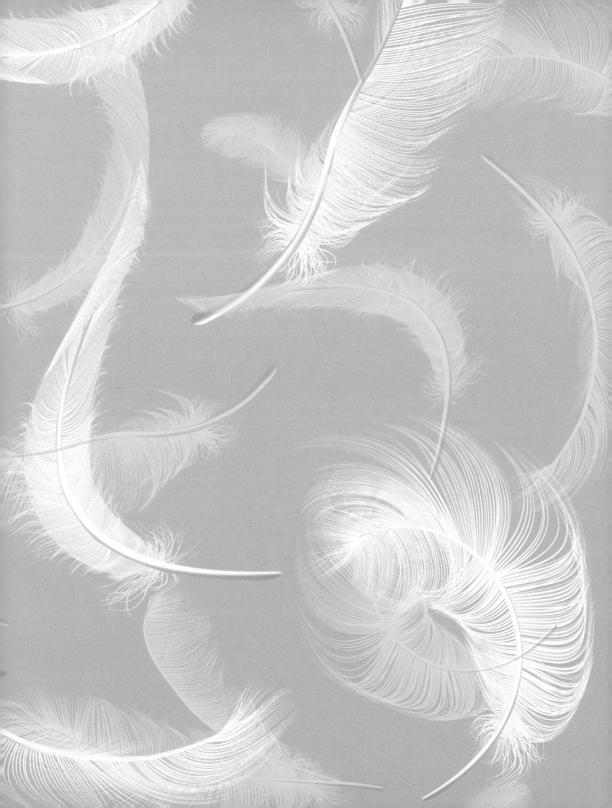

INTRODUCTION

Sleeping is an activity that we spend an enormous portion of our lives doing and, although everyone knows that it is good for us, many of us find it difficult to get good-quality sleep on a regular basis. Given today's hectic and fast-paced world, it's hardly surprising that there seem to be hundreds of barriers to sleeping well – from streetlights and noisy neighbours to worries about tomorrow's work schedule or keeping up with the latest TV boxset.

As well as sleep, dreaming is an important component of our nocturnal lives. Dreaming helps us to make sense of the day's activities, and can also provide us with the tools and symbols to resolve our problems and understand our behaviour and relationships.

This night-time journal is for anyone who wants to replace hours of tossing and turning with the joy of waking up bright-eyed and bushy-tailed, refreshed and bounding with energy and enthusiasm for the day ahead. By completing the exercises in each chapter, you'll discover patterns in your behaviour and environment that will help you improve the quality of your sleep, and you'll learn to analyze your dreams and unlock the treasure trove of wondrous information that is hidden within your subconscious.

By the time you reach the end of the journal, you should feel healthier, fitter, happier and more positive when you get out of bed each morning, and you'll have a much greater insight into the meaning of your dreams. We hope that the exercises and information in the pages that follow will help you to sleep well and dream well. Now, let's begin...

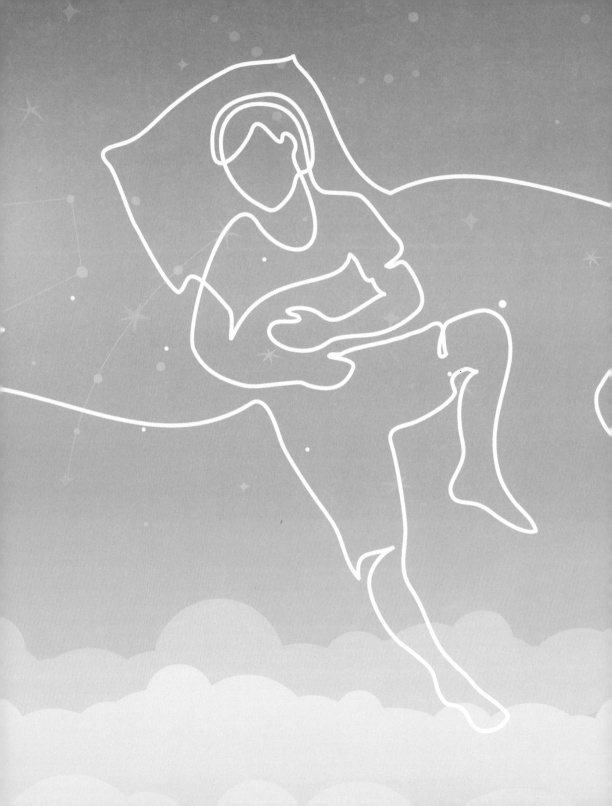

Part one
SLEEP WELL

Getting a good night's sleep is critical for our health and well-being, helping our bodies to repair themselves and also allowing our minds to rest and prepare for the day ahead. The first part of this journal looks at the benefits of sleep, and provides tips, techniques and exercises for improving your sleep. There is guidance on keeping a sleep journal, optimizing your bedroom environment, relaxing and meditating before bed, and how to get into a healthy night-time routine. By the end, you'll be looking forward to bedtime every night and replacing restlessness with blissful slumbers.

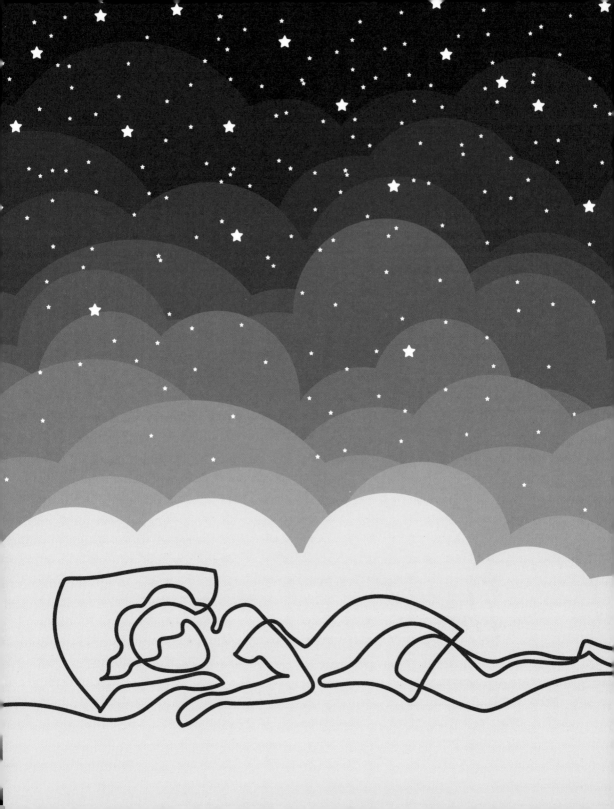

The process of sleeping

Why do we sleep?

We spend up to a third of our lives asleep and, when you think about it, lying unconscious for eight hours every night is quite a strange thing to do. Furthermore, it must've been dangerous for our ancestors, who would have been vulnerable to attack from predators while sleeping. So, like all our behaviour, there must be evolutionary advantages to sleep.

In fact, it is thought that sleep is just as necessary for our survival as eating and exercise. It allows our bodies – and in particular our brains – to recover from the day's activities. As a kind of 'clearing house', sleep strengthens important connections in the brain and removes less important ones, helping us to process our experiences and memories. It also helps with essential physiological functions, such as maintaining our immune system and regulating our metabolic function.

Getting a good night's sleep is actually one of the best things we can do if we want to be healthier, stop emotional eating and exercise better. We know this because of what happens when we don't get enough sleep: poor sleep adversely affects our brain function, immune system, hormones and exercise performance, and it can cause weight gain and increase the likelihood of disease.

Therefore, sleep is crucial for both our physical and mental well-being.

Stages of Sleep

Sleep happens in cycles, and these are repeated several times during the night – typically four or five cycles per night. Dreaming tends to happen during rapid eye movement (REM) sleep.

STAGE 1

When we initially fall asleep, we experience a very light 'catnap' sleep from which it is easy to awaken. We have slow eye movements and our muscles become relaxed. Some people have muscle spasms or jerks at this time, or may experience the sensation of falling. Stage 1 usually lasts around 5–10 minutes.

STAGE 2

During the second stage, we move into a slightly deeper sleep from which it is more difficult to awaken. Our eyes stop moving, our body temperature decreases and our heart rate begins to slow. This stage is sometimes known as non-rapid eye movement (NREM) sleep. It lasts around 10–25 minutes.

STAGE 3

The third stage is a deeper form of NREM sleep. This is the most restorative and deepest stage of sleep, from which it is difficult to awaken. Sleepwalking and sleep talking can occur, and this stage lasts around 20–40 minutes.

STAGE 4

During the fourth stage of sleep, our body becomes immobilized, REM occurs, our heart rate quickens, our blood pressure rises and our brain activity increases. It is during this stage that dreams occur. We can be awakened more easily during REM sleep, but being woken can leave us feeling disoriented and groggy. REM sleep lasts around 10 minutes during the first cycle, but gets progressively longer as the night goes on.

Sleeping positions

While we're asleep, we typically move around and adopt several different postures, but most people prefer one of three positions when falling asleep: side, front or back. It's a personal choice for everyone and there's no 'correct' way of positioning yourself when sleeping, but it's worth bearing in mind that each position exerts different pressures on our bodies.

Lying on your side can put pressure on your spine. It helps to place a pillow under your waist or, if your knees are bent, place a pillow between them. This keeps your spine in a straight line.

Lying on your front can put pressure on your neck and spine, and cause muscular pain or discomfort. This can be alleviated by placing a pillow beneath your chest, to keep your neck aligned with your spine.

Lying on your back can also put pressure on your neck and spine, so make sure your pillow is supportive enough to keep your head and neck aligned with your spine. You might like to experiment with different types of pillow, such as hypoallergenic, ergonomic or memory foam. The size of your pillow can also make a difference.

Which position do you prefer sleeping in?

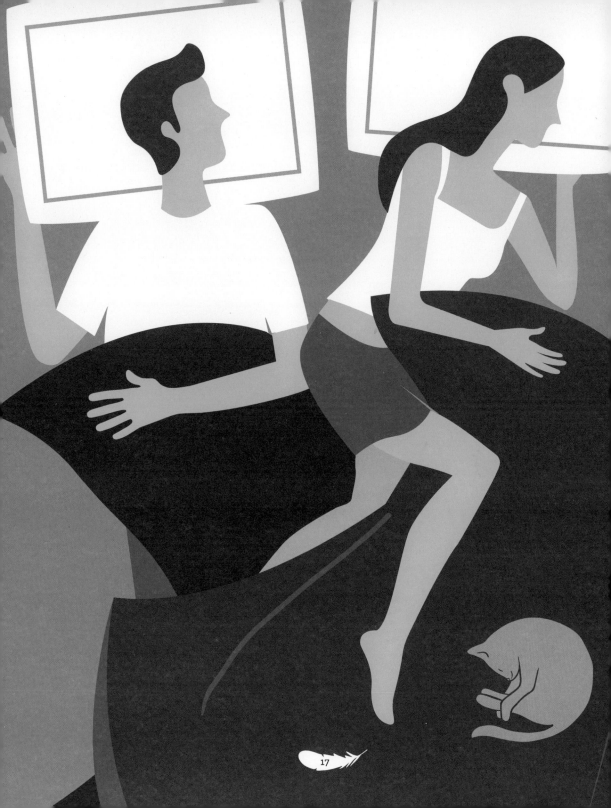

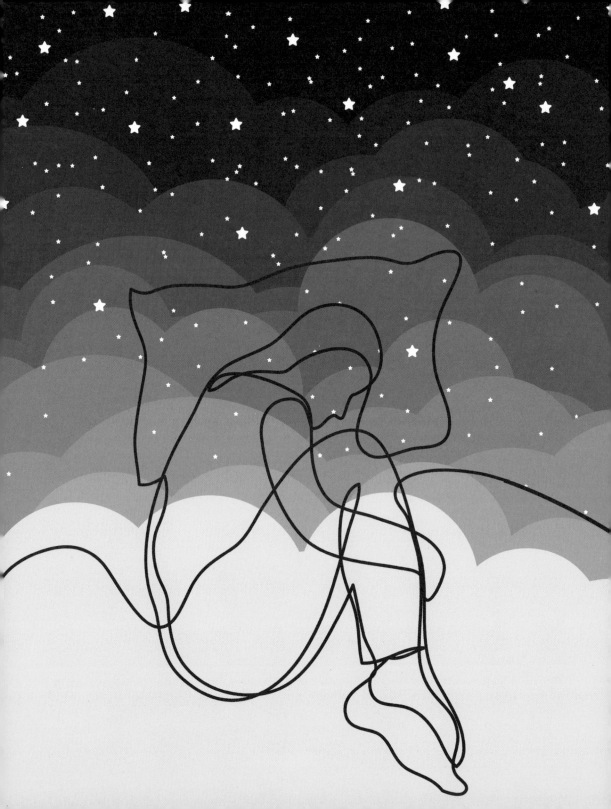

Sleep and health

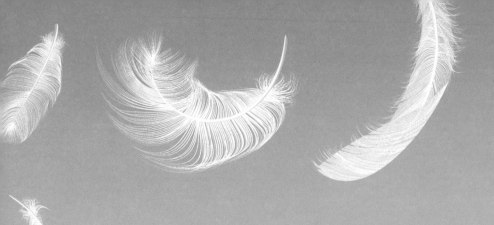

Health benefits of sleep

While we sleep, our body is actually hard at work, both physically and mentally.

We use the recuperation time to rebuild muscle tissue and cleanse harmful substances from our bodies. Sleep keeps the heart healthy by lowering blood pressure. It regulates our production of insulin, which reduces the chances of getting diabetes. It keeps our immune system strong by detecting and destroying foreign invaders in the cells; people who sleep fewer than seven hours per night, for example, are three times more likely to come down with a cold. The changes in hormone levels that occur during sleep suppress hunger, so sleep also regulates how we use food for energy and actually helps us to maintain a healthy body weight.

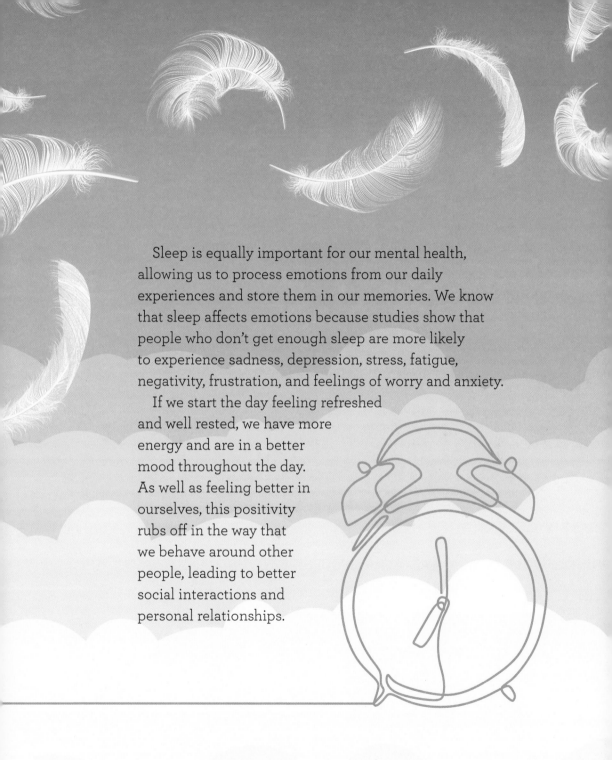

Sleep is equally important for our mental health, allowing us to process emotions from our daily experiences and store them in our memories. We know that sleep affects emotions because studies show that people who don't get enough sleep are more likely to experience sadness, depression, stress, fatigue, negativity, frustration, and feelings of worry and anxiety.

If we start the day feeling refreshed and well rested, we have more energy and are in a better mood throughout the day. As well as feeling better in ourselves, this positivity rubs off in the way that we behave around other people, leading to better social interactions and personal relationships.

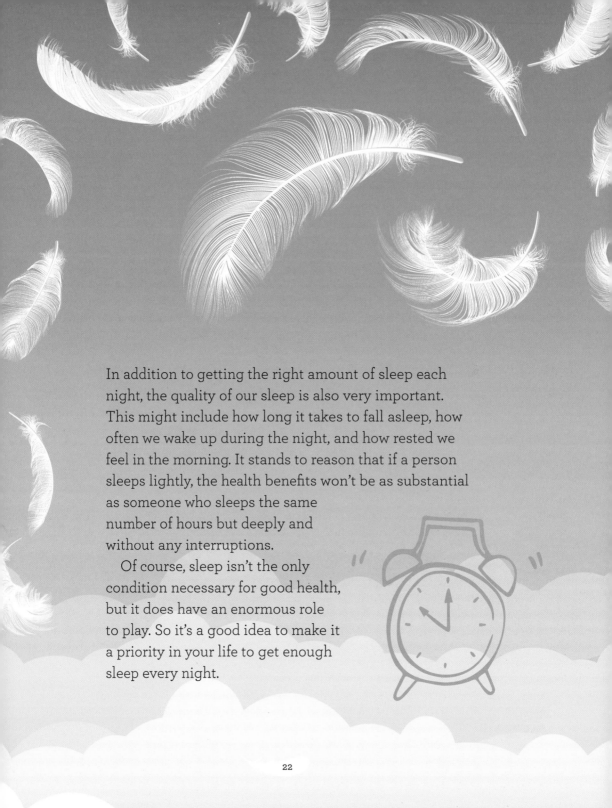

In addition to getting the right amount of sleep each night, the quality of our sleep is also very important. This might include how long it takes to fall asleep, how often we wake up during the night, and how rested we feel in the morning. It stands to reason that if a person sleeps lightly, the health benefits won't be as substantial as someone who sleeps the same number of hours but deeply and without any interruptions.

Of course, sleep isn't the only condition necessary for good health, but it does have an enormous role to play. So it's a good idea to make it a priority in your life to get enough sleep every night.

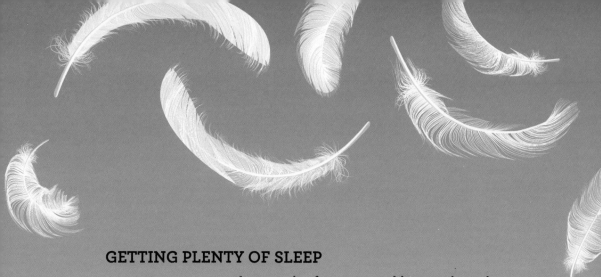

GETTING PLENTY OF SLEEP

- Improves cardiovascular function and lowers the risk of heart disease.
- Maintains healthy muscles.
- Decreases blood sugar levels and lowers the risk of type 2 diabetes.
- Strengthens the immune system.
- Decreases inflammation.
- Suppresses hunger and regulates the appetite, preventing weight gain.
- Forms connections in the brain that help us to process and remember information.
- Makes us happier and in a more positive mood.
- Improves mental health.
- Reduces stress levels.
- Improves concentration and problem-solving skills.
- Benefits social interactions and relationships.

EXERCISE:

Health goals

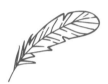

Think about how you feel now – your sense of wellbeing, your level of fitness, how often you are ill, your weight, your mood, your stress and concentration levels, and how you interact with other people. Use the space opposite to list the ways you'd like to improve your health, physically, mentally and emotionally.

1. _____

2. _____

3. _____

4. _____

5. _____

6. _____

7. _____

8. _____

9. _____

10. _____

11. _____

12. _____

13. _____

14. _____

15. _____

16. _____

17. _____

18. _____

19. _____

20. _____

How much sleep do we need?

Different individuals need different amounts of sleep each night; some people need more sleep, some less. If we look at a few famous cases, Albert Einstein reportedly slept for 10 hours per night, while Winston Churchill only got five or six hours (plus a few power naps during the day). Margaret Thatcher slept for four hours a night on weekdays, while it's said that Leonardo da Vinci took 20-minute power naps every four hours.

The amount of sleep we need is related to our age, with children needing quite a lot more sleep than older people. Generally, most adults need around seven to nine hours of sleep per night.

SLEEP THROUGHOUT OUR LIFETIME

STAGE OF LIFE	AGE	HOURS OF SLEEP NEEDED PER NIGHT
Newborns	0–3 months	14–17 hours
Infants	4–11 months	12–15 hours
Toddlers	1–2 years	11–14 hours
Preschoolers	3–5 years	10–13 hours
School children	6–13 years	9–11 hours
Teenagers	14–17 years	8–10 hours
Adults	18–64 years	7–9 hours
Older adults	65+ years	7–8 hours

As well as quantity of sleep, it's important to take sleep quality into account. If you sleep for enough hours but your quality of sleep is poor, you'll still feel tired in the morning. Conversely, if you have good-quality sleep, you may be able to get away with fewer hours of sleep.

If you think for a moment about how you're feeling during the day, you'll probably know instinctively whether you're getting enough sleep. You should feel energetic and alert in the daytime; if you feel fatigued and sluggish, you probably need more sleep or better-quality sleep.

EXERCISE:
My sleep journal

	Time you woke up	How do you feel today?	Time and duration of any daytime naps	Time to bed
MONDAY				
TUESDAY				
WEDNESDAY				
THURSDAY				
FRIDAY				
SATURDAY				
SUNDAY				

For one week, keep a record of how many hours of sleep you get each night, and whether you woke up during the night. Include notes about your emotions – do you feel energized, refreshed and in a positive mood, or tired, sluggish and in a negative mood? At the end of the week, look back over your notes. Have any noticeable patterns emerged?

Estimated time you fell asleep	Number of times you woke up during the night, and duration	When you woke up, what were your thoughts and emotions?	Total number of hours spent asleep

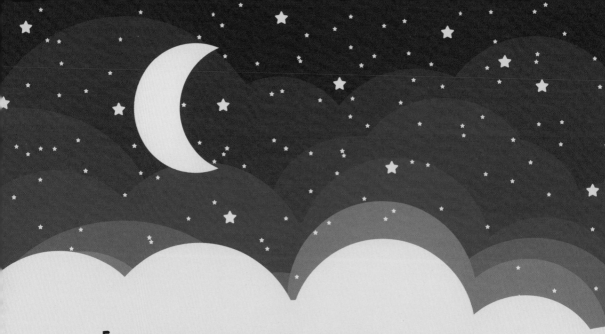

Effects of sleep deprivation

· · · · · · · · · · · · · ☾ · · · · · · · · · · · ·

If you've ever spent the night staring at the ceiling and unable to fall asleep, you're not alone. At various times in our lives we've probably all experienced bouts of insomnia, and we know that it makes us feel awful the next morning. But sleep deprivation is more than just a mild inconvenience; it's actually a very serious health risk, affecting both our physical and mental well-being.

Poor-quality sleep or not getting enough sleep increases the risk of chronic conditions such as heart disease, weight gain and type 2 diabetes. It can cause raised blood pressure and a weakened immune system, as well as poor balance and coordination, which may in turn result in falls or other accidents. Sadly, we hear all too often about road accidents caused by drivers falling asleep at the wheel.

Sleep deprivation also depletes energy and lowers libido, and is even associated with an increased chance of developing Alzheimer's disease,

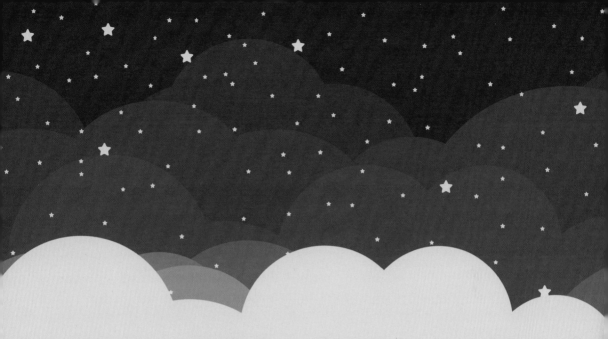

possibly because the body is not getting enough time to clear harmful waste products from the brain.

As well as these physical effects, sleep deprivation has a wide range of mental and emotional consequences. It affects our mood, making us feel more negative and short-tempered. It curbs our creativity and makes us less productive, and it impairs our concentration, problem-solving and decision-making abilities – so we're actually less effective in all areas of our lives when we're sleep-deprived, from doing a day's work to going to the supermarket.

The good news is that whatever the cause of your sleep deprivation – a stressful job, shift work, family issues, a sleep disorder or just getting into a bad habit – it's never too late to address the problem and improve your sleep.

Sleep disorders

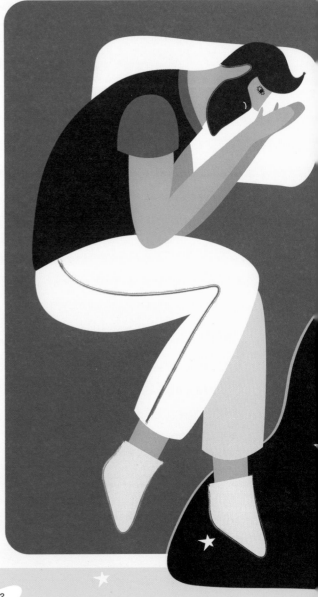

There are several sleep disorders that affect how we sleep. If any of these start to interfere with your daily life, it's a good idea to talk to your doctor so that you can get the most appropriate treatment.

Insomnia is an inability to fall asleep or stay asleep; it feels like you can't switch your brain off at night. There are many possible causes, such as anxiety, depression, stress, jet lag, caffeine, medications or an underlying health condition. Whatever the cause of your sleeplessness, learning how to relax and meditate might be your first course of action.

Sleep apnoea is a disorder in which your breathing briefly and repeatedly stops while you're asleep, causing you to wake up frequently. The pauses in breathing last for about 10 seconds, and are caused by the muscles at the back of the throat failing to keep the airway open. This condition results in loud snoring, making it very difficult for anyone to sleep next to a sufferer. Improving your physical fitness can help, as well as taking a short nap in the mid-afternoon, but you should see your doctor to get a proper diagnosis and the correct treatment.

Restless leg syndrome (RLS) is characterized by an overwhelming urge to move your legs (or occasionally arms) at night when you are at rest. It is sometimes accompanied by unpleasant crawling or aching sensations, and can be profoundly disturbing. Regular exercise, quitting smoking and adopting good sleeping habits can minimize the symptoms.

Narcolepsy is a rare sleep disorder in which a person suddenly falls asleep at inappropriate times during the day; it can happen in the middle of a conversation or while driving a car. It is thought to be caused by the lack of a brain chemical which regulates sleeping and wakefulness, and there is no known cure. However, observing a strict routine at bedtime and taking short naps evenly spaced throughout the day can help.

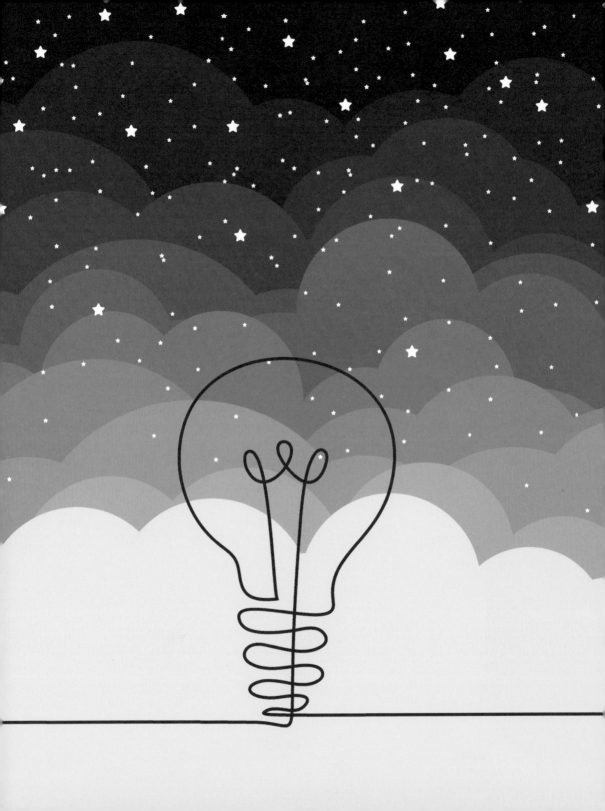

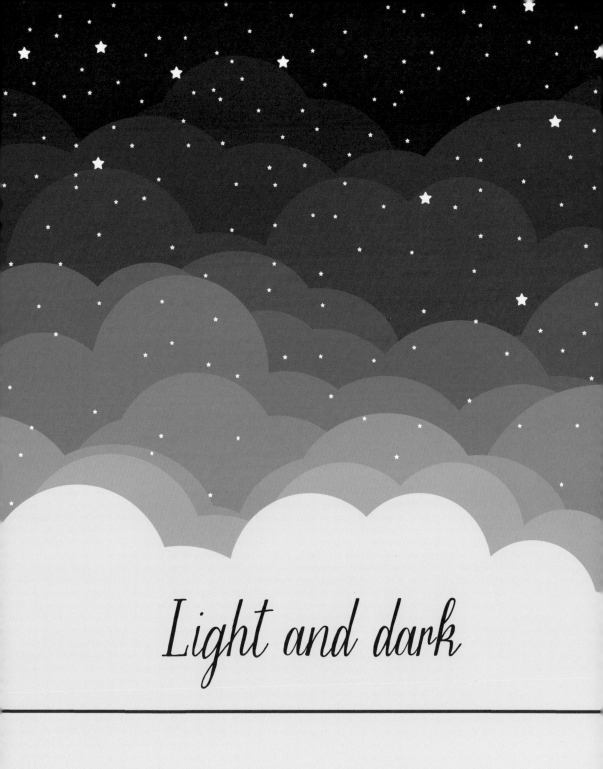

Light and dark

Daytime Light

Light levels have a very strong effect on sleep. Humans are 'diurnal', which means we're active during the day and inactive at night, and this biological predisposition makes it natural for us to be awake when it's light and asleep when it's dark.

Supporting the commonly held view that sunshine makes us happy, it's been shown in imaging experiments that the brain is more active when the ambient light is bright. Our cognitive function is also better in bright light, and sleep studies have shown that exposure to light during the day keeps energy levels high and improves one's mood.

Ideally, we're exposed to bright light first thing in the morning – our bodies and minds wake up and we feel alert when the sun streams through the bedroom window. The daytime light then helps us to recognize the contrasting evening darkness later on. This regulates our sleep/wake cycle and helps us to fall asleep when the sun goes down. Our bodies release a hormone called melatonin at night, but this only happens after we've been exposed to light during the day.

For this reason, spending time outdoors in natural light during the day helps us to fall asleep at night. Note that natural light (and that includes overcast days too) is more than a hundred times better than the brightest of lightbulbs. This exposure, contrasted with darkness at night, helps us to calibrate our internal body clock so that we know when it's time to sleep.

So, even if you work indoors, try to go outside for an hour at lunchtime. The light will improve your mood and productivity while you're awake, and it will also help you to sleep better at night.

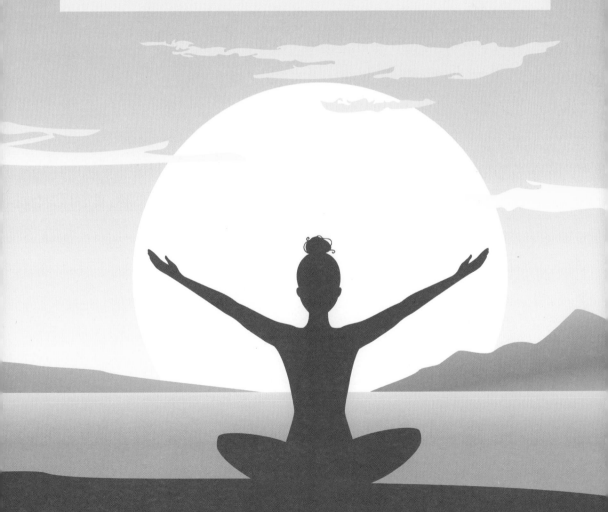

Night-time Light

The advent of electricity in the 20th century revolutionized modern life in countless wonderful ways, but unfortunately it also had a very undesirable effect on our sleeping patterns. Artificial light – in all its forms – wreaks havoc with our biological rhythms, making it much harder for us to fall asleep and get good-quality sleep.

Essentially, light signals to our body that we should be awake. So if we are exposed to light at night-time, we're confused about whether we should be awake or asleep. Rule number one is, therefore: don't sleep with the light on.

This problem is particularly marked in the case of blue light, because our eyes are especially sensitive to blue light. During the day, blue light (either natural or artificial) boosts our mood and keeps our attention levels high, helping us to stay alert. But being exposed to blue light at night disrupts our sleep cycle and prevents the right amount of melatonin from being produced in our bodies.

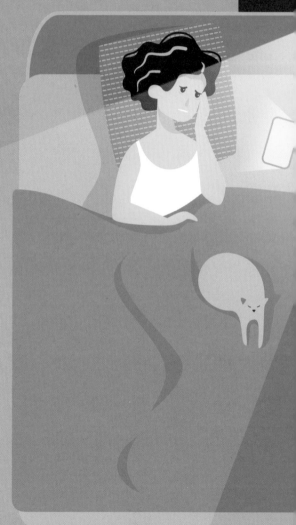

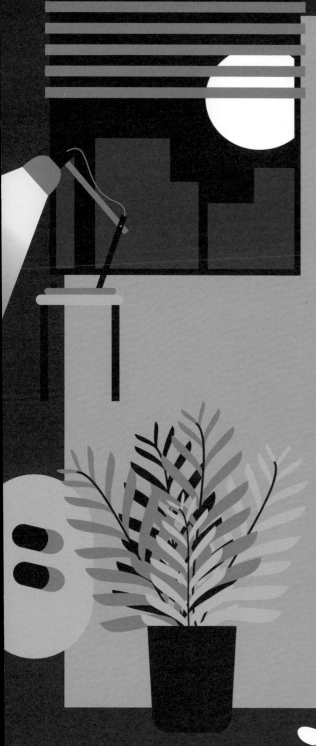

DEVICES THAT EMIT BLUE LIGHT

The following digital devices emit blue light, and should be avoided for at least an hour before bedtime:

- Televisions.
- Computers.
- Phones.
- iPads and other tablets.
- LED lights.
- Fluorescent lights.

Watching your favourite boxset on TV, checking your social media apps or reading an eBook on your iPad are among the worst things you can do just before bedtime, if you want to sleep well.

Fortunately, it is now possible to buy laptops, phones and tablets that have a blue light shield that filters out the blue light from the device. If you have the option, always put your device into 'night mode' when using it before bed. Then, 60 minutes before you want to go to sleep, switch everything off.

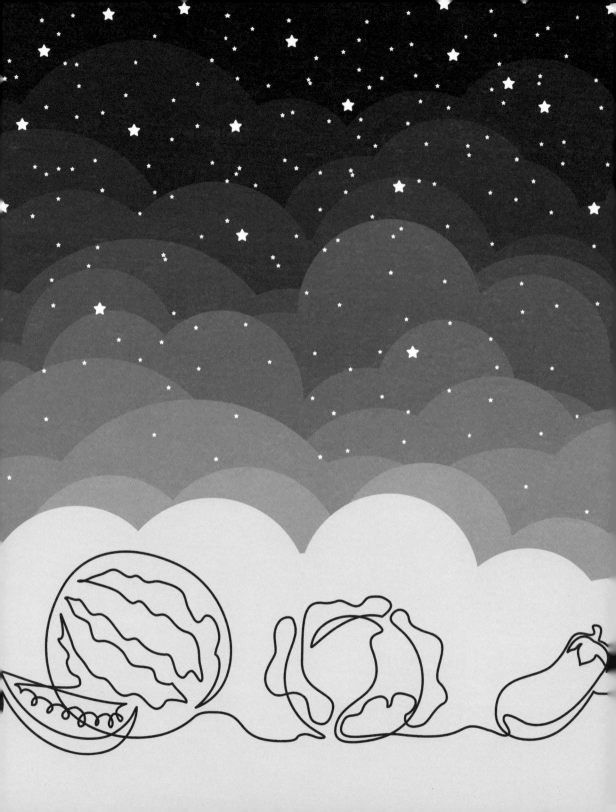

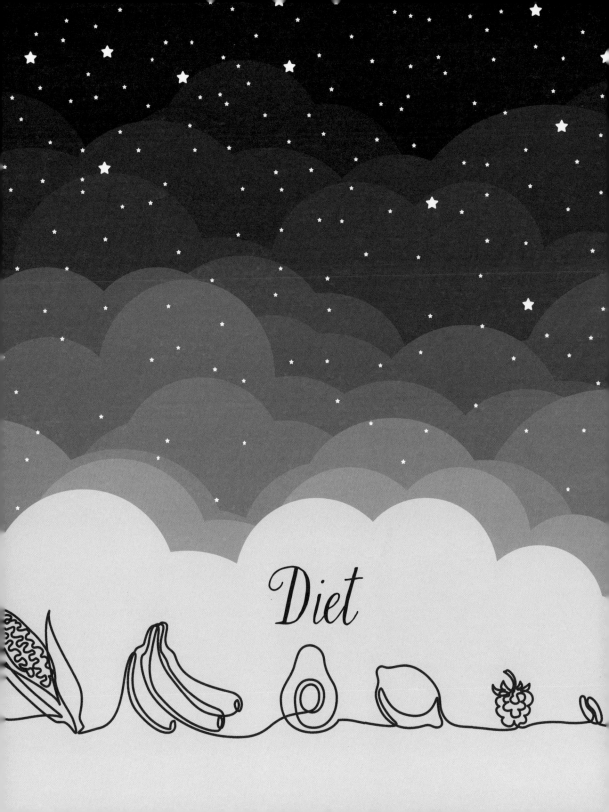

Diet

Foods

························ 🌙 ························

There are quite a few foods that are believed to promote good sleep, and it's worth bearing the properties of the following in mind when planning your evening meals.

Almonds are a source of both melatonin and magnesium. The former is the hormone that regulates sleep, while the latter is a mineral that reduces inflammation. Try eating a handful before bedtime and see whether you have a better night's sleep.

Turkey is thought to improve sleep quality because it contains the amino acid tryptophan, which increases the production of melatonin. The protein in turkey also induces a feeling of tiredness.

Kiwi fruit contains antioxidants and is good for digestive health. It also contains serotonin, the chemical that helps to regulate sleep rhythms. Eating one or two kiwi fruits before bedtime may improve sleep quality and help you to stay asleep for longer.

Fatty fish such as salmon, tuna, trout and mackerel contain a combination of omega-3 fatty acids and vitamin D. Together, these increase the production of serotonin, the brain chemical that promotes sleep.

Walnuts are a good source of the sleep-regulating hormone melatonin, and they also contain a particular omega-3 fatty acid that increases the amount of serotonin in the brain. A handful before bedtime is all you need.

Hummus contains tryptophan, which promotes sleep. Interestingly, it doesn't have to be eaten just before bedtime; eating a spoonful for lunch works just as well.

Bananas are an excellent source of vitamin B6, which converts tryptophan into serotonin. Munching on a banana before bed increases feelings of relaxation and helps you to fall asleep.

Any light snacks that contain tryptophan and calcium are good bedtime choices. Examples include a bowl of cereal, crackers and cheese, or toast with peanut butter.

FOODS TO AVOID BEFORE BEDTIME

- Spicy and high-fat foods can cause heartburn, indigestion and acid reflux, all of which are made worse by lying down.
- Foods that are high in protein cause the body to work hard at digestion instead of sleeping.
- Foods that are high in water content, such as watermelon and celery, are natural diuretics which may result in unwelcome trips to the bathroom in the middle of the night.
- Heavy meals cause the body to focus on digestion instead of sleep. It's best not to eat a heavy meal late at night; try a lighter snack instead.

DRINKS

It's calming and relaxing to enjoy a warm drink before bed, and there are certain drinks with proven soporific properties.

Warm milk contains four sleep-inducing compounds – tryptophan, calcium, vitamin D and melatonin – so there are good scientific reasons why it's a traditional bedtime drink for both children and adults alike.

Chamomile tea lessens the effects of anxiety and depression, and contains antioxidants that reduce inflammation. It also contains apigenin, an antioxidant that makes us feel sleepy and reduces insomnia. A warm mug before retiring for the night should send you straight to sleep.

Valerian tea, made from a blend of the valerian root and hops, is an aromatic and flavourful hot drink that promotes calm and reduces feelings of anxiety. It is a powerful natural remedy that has been used to treat insomnia for centuries. Be aware, though, that it can become addictive.

Passion flower tea is a good source of the antioxidant apigenin, which has a calming effect and reduces anxiety. It also inhibits the brain chemicals that induce stress. A cup before bedtime should result in an improvement in your sleep quality.

Peppermint tea calms an upset stomach and relieves bloating, both of which aid sleep if you experience indigestion, nausea or morning sickness. It also has anti-inflammatory properties, relaxes the muscles and induces feelings of calm.

Tart cherry juice makes an excellent bedtime drink because it has a high content of melatonin, the hormone that regulates our body clock and helps us go to sleep at the right time.

DRINKS TO AVOID BEFORE SLEEP

- Any drink that contains caffeine, such as coffee, tea or hot chocolate, is to be avoided at bedtime (unless it is decaffeinated). Caffeine overactivates the mind, so it's best to have your last caffeine drink at lunchtime.
- Alcohol does not promote sleep. Although it can make you feel drowsy at first, it then stops you from entering the deeper phases of the sleep cycle.

Whichever drink you choose, don't have too much before bedtime – too much liquid will result in trips to the bathroom during the night.

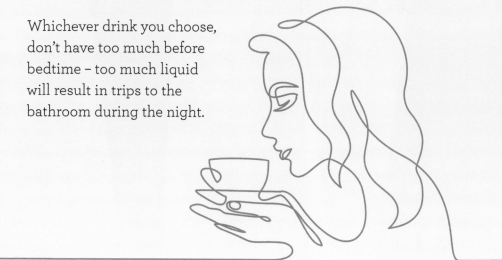

Supplements

If you ever feel the need for a little extra help in falling asleep, there are plenty of supplements on the market. They work best when used in conjunction with good sleeping habits. The following are the most common supplements for improving sleep, but it's worth noting that some of them can be found naturally in foods – so have a look at your diet before reaching for a bottle of pills.

Melatonin is a naturally occurring hormone that signals to our brain that it's time to go to sleep. Normally, levels of melatonin rise in the evening and fall in the morning, but sometimes this cycle can be disrupted, such as for shift workers or people experiencing jet lag. Melatonin supplements can help to regulate the sleep/wake cycle, in combination with sunlight exposure during the day.

Valerian root works as a sedative on the brain and nervous system, and can be taken in tablet or capsule form (as well as tea). It can help you to fall asleep faster, and also reduces the number of times you wake up during the night.

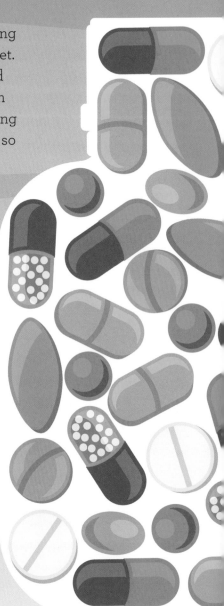

Magnesium is a mineral that increases levels of gamma-aminobutyric acid (GABA), a chemical messenger in the brain that reduces anxiety. It may be particularly effective for people who don't have enough magnesium in their diet. (Foods that contain magnesium include spinach, kale, black beans, chickpeas, kidney beans, peas, broccoli, green beans, figs, avocados, bananas, raspberries, nuts and seeds, salmon, mackerel and tuna.)

Glycine is an amino acid that has many functions relating to the immune, digestive and musculature systems, and it also quietens the brain and nervous system. As a supplement, it can reduce the time taken to fall asleep, promote deeper sleep, and lessen the symptoms of insomnia. It does all of this by lowering body temperature and increasing serotonin levels. (Foods which contain glycine include spinach, kale, cabbage, beans, bananas, kiwi fruit, eggs, bone broth, meat, poultry and fish.)

Ginkgo biloba comes from the dried green leaves of the ginkgo tree, and is used for relaxation and alleviating the symptoms of stress and anxiety. It can be taken as a liquid extract, capsule or tablet.

Cannabidiol (CBD) oil comes from the cannabis or hemp plant, and has been steadily gaining attention in recent years. It does not give you a 'high', but it can decrease chronic pain, reduce anxiety and depression, improve the symptoms of Parkinson's disease and promote the REM stage of sleep. As a bedtime drink, the dosage can be mixed with a few drops of valerian tincture and a cup of tart cherry juice.

EXERCISE:
My food and drink journal

	Breakfast	Mid-morning	Lunch	Afternoon
MONDAY				
TUESDAY				
WEDNESDAY				
THURSDAY				
FRIDAY				
SATURDAY				
SUNDAY				

For a week, list all your foods, drinks and supplements. Each morning, write down how well you slept the previous night. Can you see any interesting patterns?

Dinner	Bedtime	Describe your quality of sleep

EXERCISE:

Diet goals

Here we're not worried about diet in the sense of what to eat to lose weight, but more the diet to follow to help you sleep well. Using your food journal on pages 48-9, identify the foods and drinks that you had when you had a good night's sleep. List them opposite, and then add the foods and drinks you've not tried but think you might like that are given as good sleep promoters on pages 42-5. Experiment with your list until you find the ideal combination for a restful sleep.

Foods and drinks when you had a
good night's sleep

Foods and drinks to try

_____

_____

_____

_____

_____

_____

_____

_____

_____

_____

_____

_____

_____

_____

_____

_____

_____

_____

_____

_____

_____

_____

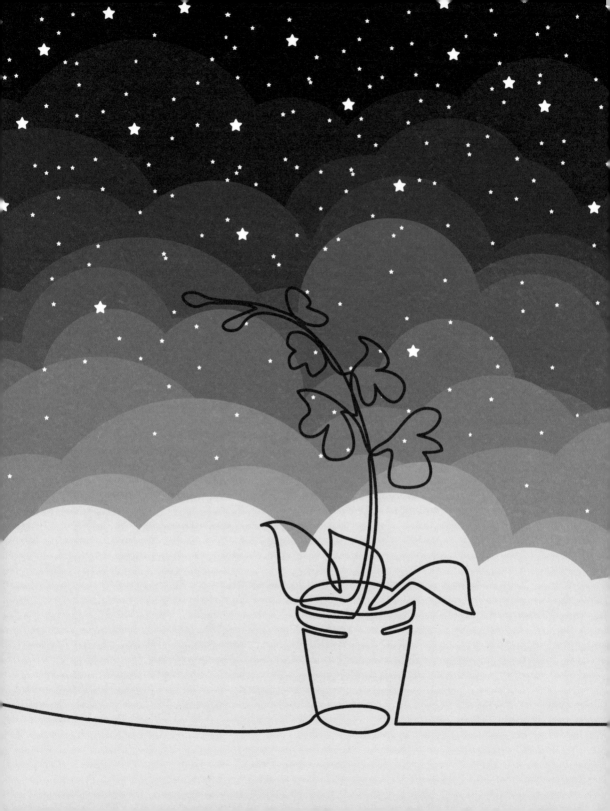

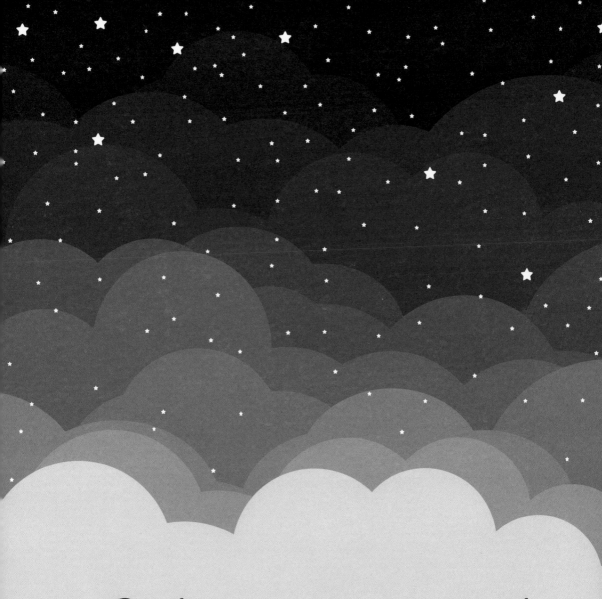

Bedroom environment

OPTIMIZE YOUR BEDROOM ENVIRONMENT

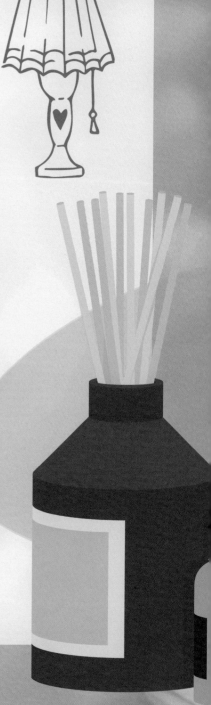

Your bedroom is where you spend a third of your life sleeping, so it makes sense to plan its features carefully and think about how to make it conducive to sleep.

Keep your bedroom dark – even a glimpse of a streetlight or the moon can disrupt your sleep. You can achieve complete darkness by covering your windows with blackout curtains, shutters or shades, or you could try wearing an eye mask. A dimmer switch is also a good way of gradually darkening the bedroom each evening. This allows your body to wind down naturally and get ready for sleep. If you do need a light source at night – for example, in a child's bedroom – use a nightlight with a red bulb, and put it in a hallway just outside the room.

Make sure your bedroom is the right temperature for sleep. This is ideally quite cool: around 15.5–19.5°C (60–67°F) for adults, or 18–21°C (65–70°F) for babies. Our bodies cool down as we fall asleep, and a cooler environment helps us to do this.

Try using scent as a sedative. The aroma of lavender is known to improve sleep quality, either in its dried form or as an essential oil. There are plenty of soporific scents you can experiment with, including vanilla, valerian extract, clary sage, sweet marjoram, sandalwood, juniper, chamomile, jasmine, rose, lemon, bergamot and frankincense. Which aroma do you like best?

Soothing music or natural background sound such as rainfall or white noise can have a powerful effect on our mood and nervous system: it can slow our heart rate and breathing, lower our blood pressure and help our muscles relax. Choose a type of music or sound that you enjoy, and incorporate it into your sleep routine. The benefits grow with time; your body gets into the habit of falling asleep when you're exposed to a relaxing soundtrack every night. Whatever sound you choose, set it on an automatic timer so that you don't have to worry about waking up to turn it off.

If unwanted noise from the neighbours or street traffic is a problem, consider soundproofing your bedroom walls, windows, ceiling and floor. There are many ways of doing this, such as using acoustic foam, double-glazing and installing carpet or rugs. Even adding a few paintings or putting up bookshelves can help. You might also try wearing ear plugs.

BEDDING AND SLEEPWEAR

What you sleep on and what you wear to bed have a huge influence on your sleep quality. Everyone is different, but there are a few important things to consider when choosing your bedding and sleepwear.

Your mattress needs to support your spine and reduce the pressure points on your body. If it's too soft, you'll sink down; if it's too hard, you'll have too much pressure on your lower back, shoulders and head. Many experts recommend replacing your mattress about every eight years.

Experiment to find the type of pillow you like best. Some people prefer very soft pillows; others prefer ergonomic or memory foam pillows.

Choose natural, breathable fibres such as cotton, wool, down, linen or silk for your sheets and bedding, and also for your sleepwear. Even the colour can help you sleep better, so choose something soothing.

Many people find that having some weight on their body helps them fall asleep – a heavy blanket can be comforting. Having said that, decide whether you want to share your bed with your pets. Note that once a cat or dog is allowed to sleep on your bed a few times, it becomes almost impossible to stop them.

Last but not least, wear socks! It is thought that warming your feet allows your internal body temperature to drop, which in turn facilitates sleep.

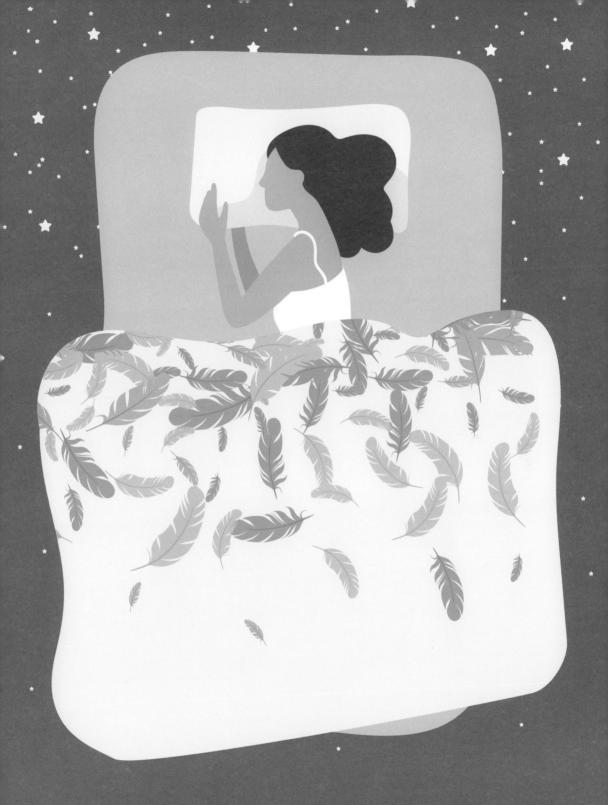

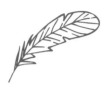

EXERCISE:
My bedroom

Go into your bedroom and look around.

In what ways could you improve your sleep environment?

_____

_____

_____

Is your bedroom dark? If not, what could you change?

_____

_____

_____

What temperature is your bedroom at night?

_____

What are your favourite aromas for making you feel drowsy?

_____

_____

Do you ever listen to music or white noise at night? What kind of music or background sound do you like best?

_____

_____

How quiet is your bedroom? How could you improve it?

_____

_____

How old is your mattress? How does your back feel when you wake up each morning?

_____

_____

What do you wear to bed?

_____

_____

If you have pets, where do they sleep? Do they ever wake you up in the middle of the night? How could you improve this?

_____

_____

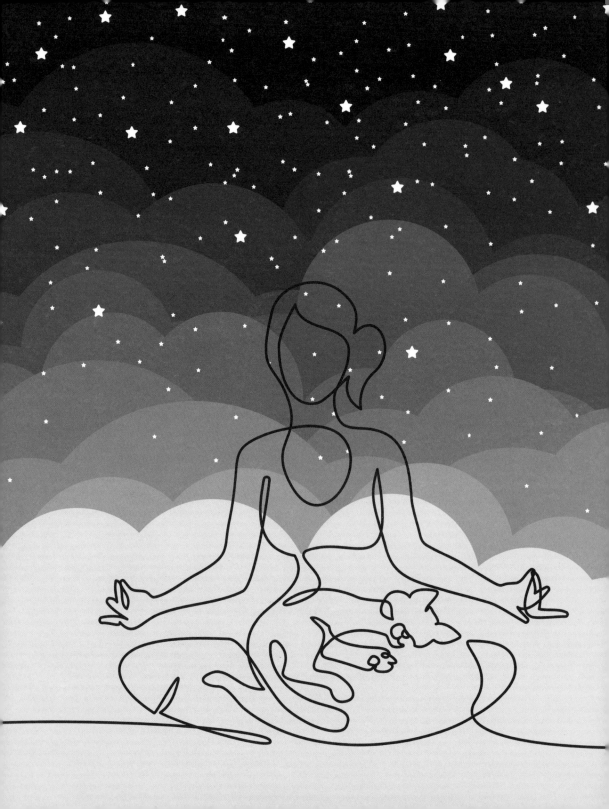

Relaxing the mind and body

MIND MANAGEMENT

Have you ever noticed that your worries seem worse at night, just when you're trying to get to sleep? It's actually very common for sleep issues and anxiety to go together – as soon as your head hits the pillow, you begin analyzing the events of the day and start worrying about what you have to do tomorrow. It's not surprising that a racing mind interferes with your ability to fall asleep.

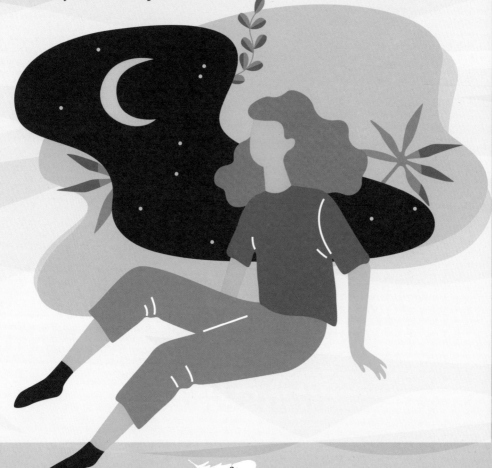

Ask yourself the following:

- Do you ever skip breakfast because you're running late?
- Do you grab a quick lunch on the go?
- Do you collapse, exhausted, in front of the TV every evening?
- Do you spend your weekends catching up on all the chores you didn't have time to do during the week?
- Do you constantly feel like you're 'behind'?

If you answer 'yes' to these sorts of questions, you're probably not giving yourself enough time to enjoy your everyday life, or even noticing how you feel during the day.

It may be time to stop and do more of the following:

Learn to say no. This may apply to many different areas of your life, from taking on extra work to attending social events. Think about whether you really want to do something; not just whether you're expected to do it.

Make time each day to slow down and pay attention to where you are now and what you're doing in the present moment.

Change your thinking. Instead of blaming yourself (or others) for past mistakes, try letting them go instead. Think constructively about how you can do things differently next time.

Keep a journal and jot down your thoughts and worries. Writing is a really good way to release stress, and can help you understand why you're feeling worried or anxious. Try writing down tomorrow's 'to do' list before you go to bed. That way your plans can spend the night on paper instead of on your mind!

RELATIONSHIPS

Our mental health is closely tied up with our personal relationships and how we connect with the people around us. Relationships with family, friends, work colleagues and the wider community all impact on our sense of well-being, and by extension, our quality of sleep.

Good relationships lead to a sense of belonging, a shared identity and community spirit. Forming healthy connections lifts us when we're down and gives us the capacity to deal with new challenges, so it makes sense to take care of our relationships in order to take care of ourselves.

Try making a weekly 'date night' to spend quality time with your partner, or schedule regular meals with a parent, sibling or friend.

Make the effort to listen more. Pay attention to what people are saying, focusing on their tone of voice and their body language.

Try to sort out disagreements or arguments quickly, instead of worrying about them at night.

Join a group of like-minded people so that you can enjoy shared activities and interests.

Spending unhurried time with people is invaluable in helping you to relax, forget your troubles and enjoy life. You will reap the benefits in your sleep quality.

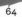

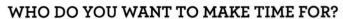

WHO DO YOU WANT TO MAKE TIME FOR?

List here the friends and family that you feel refreshed after seeing, and make a conscious effort to see more of them.

_____

_____

_____

_____

_____

_____

_____

_____

_____

_____

_____

_____

_____

_____

_____

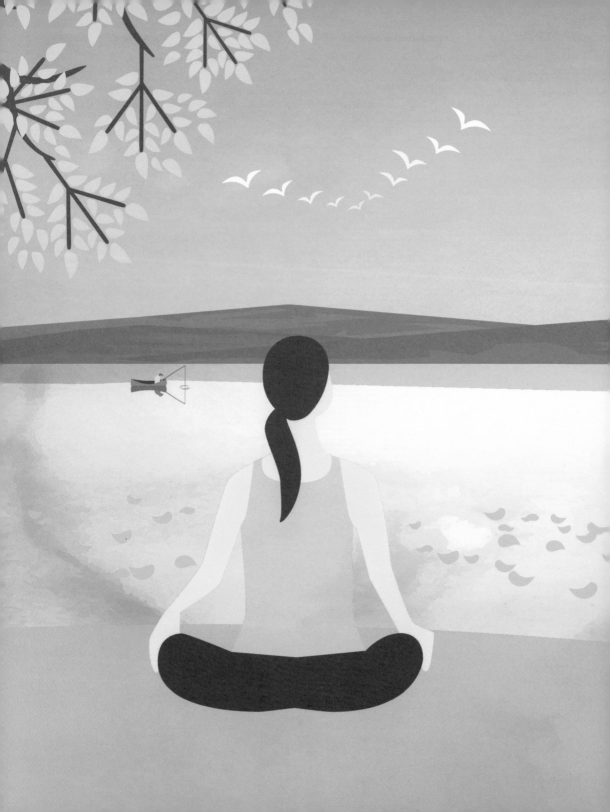

Meditation

· · · · · · · · · · · · · ☾ · · · · · · · · · · · ·

The ability to quieten your mind and prevent the intrusion of unwanted thoughts is key to falling asleep. We often find that our minds are filled with fleeting images when we go to bed, but these stray thoughts can be controlled by meditation. Meditation not only rests and relaxes the mind; it also lowers the heart rate and encourages slower breathing, allowing you to let go of the day's worries before sleep.

A good way to start meditating is to focus your thoughts on your body. If you deliberately notice the gentle, peaceful sensations that are already there, you'll soon find that your mind begins to slow down. In a nutshell, when you're focusing your attention on your body, you're not paying attention to your busy mind.

Many people find that audio recordings of guided sleep meditation are also helpful. In such recordings, a soothing voice provides step-by-step instructions to help you enter a more peaceful mindset.

Whichever method you choose, as your mind calms down, sleep will naturally follow.

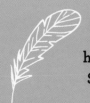

You cannot force yourself to sleep, but you can help yourself along the way by slowing your mind. Sleep is a side effect of learning how to meditate.

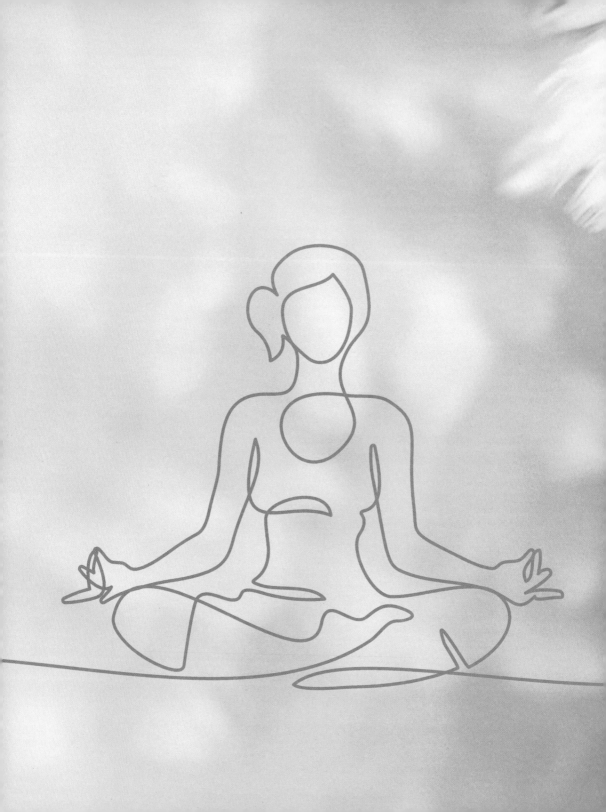

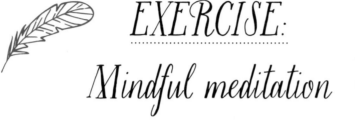

EXERCISE:
Mindful meditation

When you're lying in bed, mentally move through each part of your body, from your head down to your toes. Notice different sensations, such as tension, lightness, heaviness, tingling or temperature. As you move through each body part, imagine yourself breathing into that part and releasing any tension.

Picture your worrying thoughts moving past you like clouds floating across the sky, birds flying into the distance or leaves floating down a river. As you do this, your body will begin to relax and you will breathe more deeply.

Visualize a beautiful, peaceful scene, perhaps a place you've enjoyed visiting in the past. Try to recall as much detail as you can – for example, the colour of the sky, the feeling of warm sunshine on your face and the lightness of your mood. Visualizing a happy scene will give you a calm sense of well-being.

Relaxation

Many people think they're too busy to set aside time for relaxing, but in fact relaxation is one of the most important things we can ever do. As well as benefiting and refreshing our body, relaxation also helps us to achieve a clear and calm mind – exactly what we need when we're trying to fall asleep.

There are lots of different ways to relax:

Deep breathing allows the body to take in more oxygen. This helps to slow the heart rate, reduce blood pressure and relieve anxiety and stress.

Progressive muscle relaxation is a technique whereby each muscle of the body in turn is consciously tensed and then relaxed.

Visualization reduces intrusive thoughts by picturing a relaxing setting in our mind's eye and then focusing on the details.

Chanting is a mindfulness technique that keeps us in the present moment, helping us to quieten our thoughts. You could try a traditional mantra such as 'Om Shanti' (for peace), or make up your own.

Taking a hot bath not only feels comforting, it also aids sleep because it helps to lower body temperature. Your temperature rises when you're in the bath, and your body's response to the heat increase is to lower your internal temperature.

Having fun with family and friends or indulging in a creative hobby – in fact, doing any activity that you enjoy – is a form of relaxation that boosts your mood.

EXERCISE:

How to fall asleep in 60 seconds

Here are two methods for falling asleep quickly, the first focusing on breathing and the second on relaxing your muscles. The more you practise them, the more effective they will become.

BREATHING METHOD

While doing this exercise, hold the tip of your tongue against the roof of your mouth, just behind your two front teeth.

- Part your lips slightly and exhale through your mouth, making a whooshing sound.
- Close your mouth and inhale silently through your nose. Count to four in your head as you inhale.
- Hold your breath for seven seconds.
- Exhale for seven seconds, making another whooshing sound.
- Repeat this cycle for four full breaths, or until you fall asleep.

PROGRESSIVE MUSCLE RELAXATION METHOD

In this method, you need to tense and then relax your muscles. You should feel the tension in your body diminish as you go.

- Raise your eyebrows as high as you can, and hold for five seconds. You should feel your forehead muscles tighten. Relax your eyebrows and wait for 10 seconds. You should feel the tension drop.
- Smile widely to tighten the muscles in your cheeks. Hold for five seconds. Then relax for 10 seconds.
- Close your eyes as tightly as you can, and hold for five seconds. Then relax for 10 seconds.
- Tilt your head back so that you're looking up at the ceiling, and hold for five seconds. Then let your head come back down and relax on the pillow for 10 seconds.
- Repeat these exercises throughout your body, tensing and relaxing the muscles in your shoulders, arms, chest, abdomen, back, hips, buttocks, legs and feet.
- Let yourself fall asleep, even if you haven't finished relaxing your entire body.

Yoga and massage

The popular practice of yoga is an excellent way to wind down in preparation for sleep. It combines postures with breathing techniques, builds core strength, improves flexibility and muscle tone, and helps the mind to relax.

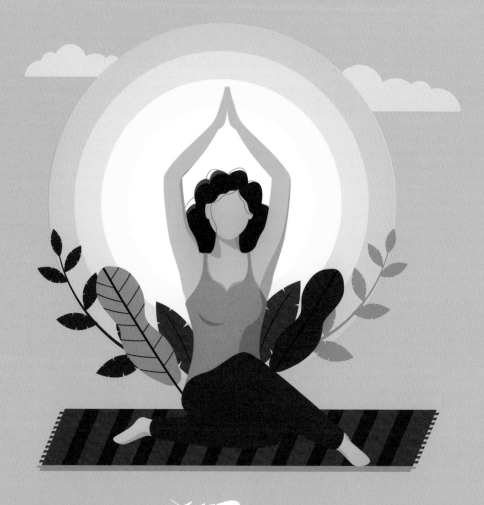

There are many resting postures and active postures that you can do, and each one involves inhaling and exhaling along with muscle stretches. Three good yoga positions to try as part of your bedtime routine are:

LEGS UP THE WALL

Lie on the floor and put your legs up the wall so that your body forms an L shape. Hold for 30 seconds and focus on your breathing.

LYING BUTTERFLY

Lie on the floor on your back and press your feet together, allowing your knees to fall to the sides.

CORPSE POSE

Lie on your back with your legs straight and your arms by your sides, palms upwards. Keep breathing slowly.

Massage is also very good for sleep, helping us to relax and feel less pain. It has been shown to boost serotonin, the 'happiness' brain chemical that regulates our sleep cycle. In fact, massage is so beneficial to sleep that some say it almost manually imposes sleep.

There are several types of massage, including Swedish massage, deep massage, sports massage and trigger point massage, or you can try self-massage to ease knots in your shoulder and neck muscles.

Positive thinking

Getting in the right mood for sleep is half the battle won, and cognitive behavioural therapy (CBT) can really help with this. Essentially, CBT helps you to replace negative thoughts with positive ones.

A typical internal conversation might go like this: 'I'm exhausted and I really need to get some sleep tonight. What time is it? I can't believe I'm not asleep yet! I've got a really big day tomorrow. If I fall asleep in the next hour, I'll get five hours. I'm so angry I'm still wide awake! If I fall asleep now, I'll get four hours.' And so on.

Another way to describe this type of conversation is a 'self-fulfilling prophesy'. You think you won't fall asleep, so you don't.

But with CBT, you can replace the negative thoughts with positivity and acceptance. For example, you might reframe your internal conversation as: 'I'm resting in bed and it feels nice. Eventually I'll fall asleep. If I have to, I can function on a little less sleep; it's not the end of the world if I don't get a full night's sleep tonight. I'll go to bed earlier tomorrow night.'

It's important to try to limit negative thoughts about sleep, because your subconscious can easily begin to associate bedtime with anxiety. By changing the narrative in your head, you can break the cycle.

Negative thought:

_____

_____

_____

Positive reframe:

_____

_____

_____

Negative thought:

_____

_____

_____

Positive reframe:

_____

_____

_____

READ A BOOK

Many of us grow up hearing bedtime stories as children, and there are scientific reasons why becoming immersed in a story just before going to sleep can enhance our relaxation and improve our quality of sleep. So don't leave bedtime books on the shelf just because you're no longer a child – there are some great benefits in reading a book before you close your eyes at night. Here are a few:

- When you're tired and stressed, a story can become a haven of calm, holding your attention and distracting you from life's stresses and worries. The narrative of the story takes your mind somewhere else, allowing you to forget your troubles for a while.
- Reading helps your muscles to relax and slows down your breathing, resulting in feelings of serenity and tranquillity.
- If you read a book every night at the same time, it creates a good bedtime routine – and keeping to a consistent sleep schedule regulates your body clock and helps you to fall asleep and stay asleep all night.

BOOK RECOMMENDATIONS

Ask your friends to recommend books that are happy and relaxing to read – so no gripping thrillers or exciting plots that will keep you awake for just one more chapter. List them here so you always know where to look for your next read.

1. _____

2. _____

3. _____

4. _____

5. _____

6. _____

7. _____

8. _____

9. _____

10. _____

11. _____

12. _____

13. _____

14. _____

15. _____

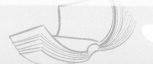

Getting out of bed in the morning

Many people find it difficult to get up when the alarm clock goes off, but there are a few things you can do to make it easier.

First, breathe slowly and deeply. With each intake of air, visualize oxygen entering your lungs and spreading to your head, body, arms, legs and toes. Rub your arms from your elbows to your wrists, to boost the flow of energy.

Stimulate the pressure points in your ears by placing your hands over your ears and rubbing them vigorously up and down 10 times.

Stimulate the pressure points in your hands by gently rubbing your palms, wrists and fingers with your thumbs.

Finally, place your hands on the lower left side of your abdomen and apply pressure while making small circular movements, gradually moving up your ribcage. Do the same on your right side. This will help to kick-start your digestive system.

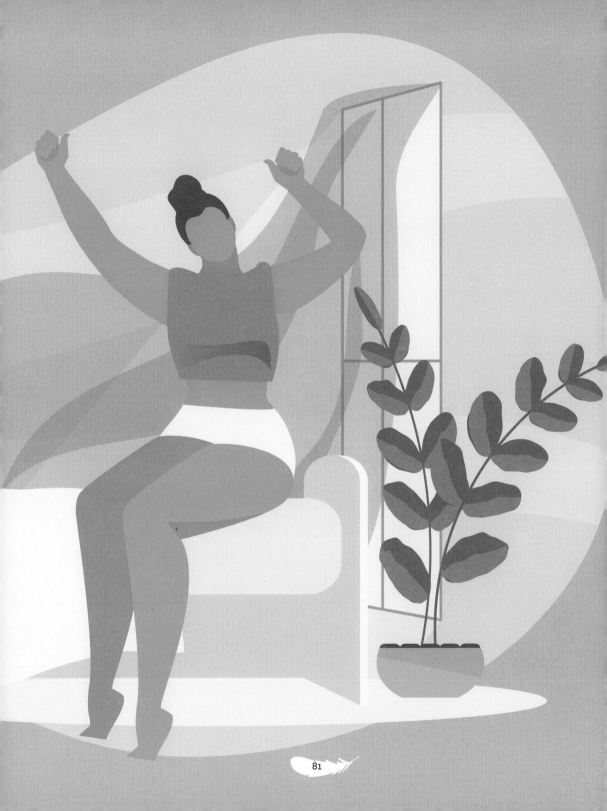

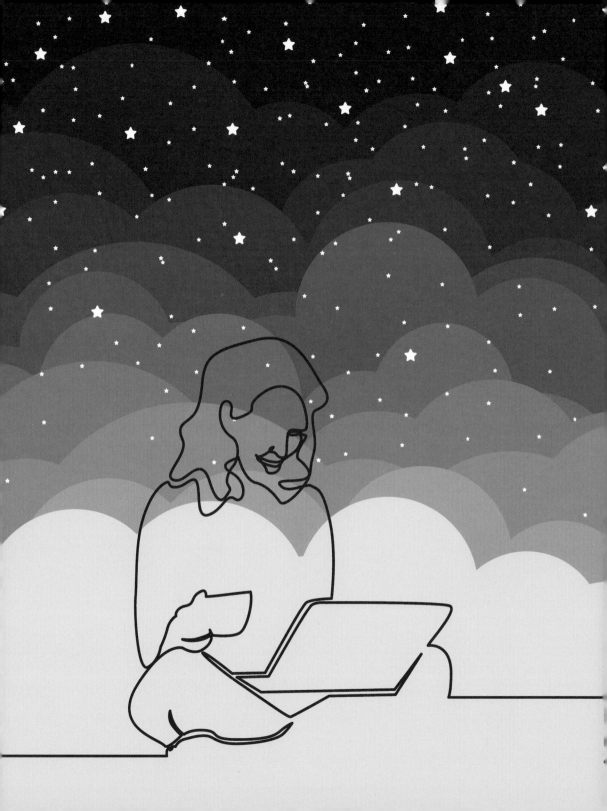

Routines

BODY CLOCK

Our sleep routine is biologically regulated by a circadian rhythm, also known as our body clock or sleep/wake cycle. All humans naturally run on a 24-hour cycle, with sunshine causing us to feel alert and darkness causing us to feel sleepy. There are variations among individuals, with some people being 'skylarks' and others being 'night owls', and also variations for different age groups, with teenagers typically sleeping longer, going to bed later and waking up later than older adults.

Our body clock works best when we stick to regular sleeping habits, but it can go wrong in certain circumstances:

- When the clocks change from daylight saving time to winter time, and vice versa.
- When we stay up later than usual.
- When we experience jet lag, caused by travelling across multiple time zones.

These sorts of problems are usually temporary, and your body will readjust its internal clock to reset the sleep/wake cycle within a few days. It may help to take short naps during the day while you're adjusting – but no more than two hours. The most important thing you can do is re-establish your bedtime routine as quickly as you can. Record your morning and evening routines opposite so you have an ideal plan to work toward.

MORNING ROUTINE

_____

_____

_____

_____

_____

_____

_____

_____

_____

_____

_____

_____

_____

_____

EVENING ROUTINE

_____

_____

_____

_____

_____

_____

_____

_____

_____

_____

_____

_____

_____

_____

Daily activity

Doing a bit of exercise every day can dramatically improve your sleep. It can increase the amount of time you spend in deep sleep and also help you to stay asleep for longer.

Being active also benefits your mental health, keeping stress and anxiety at bay. Even five minutes of exercise can trigger the anti-anxiety response in your body – and if you're feeling relaxed, you're more likely to sleep well. Exercising for 30 minutes a day is even better.

Early morning and afternoon are the best times to exercise, as this helps to regulate your body clock – your temperature goes up during exercise and then when it drops later, you're ready to sleep. It's best if you exercise outdoors, because then you'll be exposing yourself to natural light.

Try not to exercise too late in the day, as you'll raise your body temperature and keep yourself awake. Some light stretching or an evening stroll three to four hours before bedtime are fine.

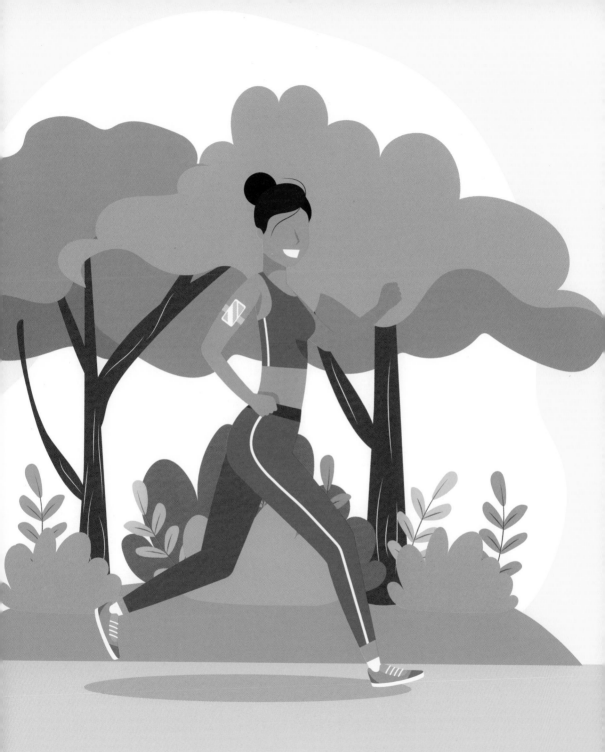

EXERCISE:
Physical exercises for improving your sleep

Here are some good activities that will help you get a better night's sleep.

Aerobic (or cardio) training such as running, brisk walking, riding a bike or swimming gets your heart rate up. Aim for 30 minutes, five days a week.

Strength exercises such as squats, lunges, sit-ups, push-ups, bicep curls and shoulder presses are good for building muscle.

Yoga and pilates not only calm the mind, they also improve circulation and muscle tone, and help to remove toxins from the body. There are lots of great exercises and positions to try, from rotating your shoulders to standing with your back against a wall and bending as far forwards as you can go.

List the exercises you'd like to try on the page opposite.

1. _____

2. _____

3. _____

4. _____

5. _____

6. _____

7. _____

8. _____

9. _____

10. _____

11. _____

12. _____

13. _____

14. _____

15. _____

16. _____

17. _____

18. _____

19. _____

20. _____

EXERCISE:
My daily activity routine

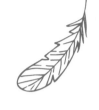

	Activities during the day	Time of day for each activity
MONDAY		
TUESDAY		
WEDNESDAY		
THURSDAY		
FRIDAY		
SATURDAY		
SUNDAY		

Keep a weekly diary recording your bedtime routine and you'll soon discover how much it varies throughout the week. Doing some exercise during the day and sticking to a regular bedtime schedule at night will help you to fall asleep more quickly and stay asleep throughout the night.

Number of minutes spent exercising	Time to bed	Describe your quality of sleep

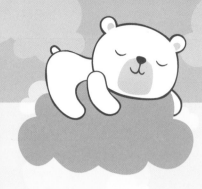

Tips for getting kids to bed

It is often difficult to get children into bed – they might be overexcited, overtired or not tired enough, or they may be stressed or trying to assert their need for independence. Whatever the situation, there are several things that you can incorporate into a child's night-time routine to help get them to sleep.

First, set a bedtime that is appropriate for the age of the child (see pages 26–7), and be consistent. Set a wake-up time as well.

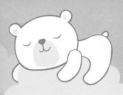
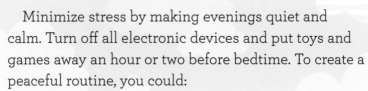

Minimize stress by making evenings quiet and calm. Turn off all electronic devices and put toys and games away an hour or two before bedtime. To create a peaceful routine, you could:

- Dim the lights.
- Give your child a small cup of warm milk.
- Play gentle, soothing music.
- Have your child take a warm bath.
- Talk in a calm voice.
- Ask your child to put on their pyjamas and brush their teeth.
- Sing a lullaby or read a bedtime story.
- Provide a teddy bear or soft toy to cuddle.
- Kiss your child goodnight.

If you do these things every night at the same time and in the same order, your child will soon expect what's coming next and will automatically start to feel sleepy when the routine begins.

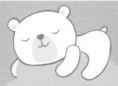

POWER NAPPING

· · · · · · · · · · · · · · ☾ · · · · · · · · · · · · · · · ·

If your sleep routine ever gets disturbed, a short power nap can help to recharge your batteries. It certainly worked for Leonardo da Vinci, Albert Einstein, Winston Churchill and President John F. Kennedy, and it's common practice in warm Mediterranean countries.

The key to a successful power nap is to doze for about 20 minutes. If you sleep any longer, you'll go into deep sleep mode and will feel even worse afterwards. The idea is to drift off from Stage 1 sleep to Stage 2 sleep (see pages 14–15), then wake up feeling refreshed and alert for the rest of your day.

Find a comfortable chair where you won't be disturbed; this could be at your desk, in your car or at home. Recline or put your head down and set an alarm to wake you 20 minutes later. Play some white noise or wear noise-cancelling headphones, if you have them, then close your eyes.

The best time for a power nap is between lunch and 3 o'clock in the afternoon, when we're digesting our food. At this time, our bodies produce insulin which triggers our sleep hormones and makes us feel drowsy.

Paradoxically, it's actually a good idea to drink a cup of coffee just before a power nap. This is because it takes 20 minutes for the caffeine to be absorbed into the body, so once your nap is over, the caffeine will kick in and make you feel alert.

Note that power naps don't suit everybody. If you have insomnia or a sleep disorder you won't feel better after a power nap, so rule those out before taking naps during the day.

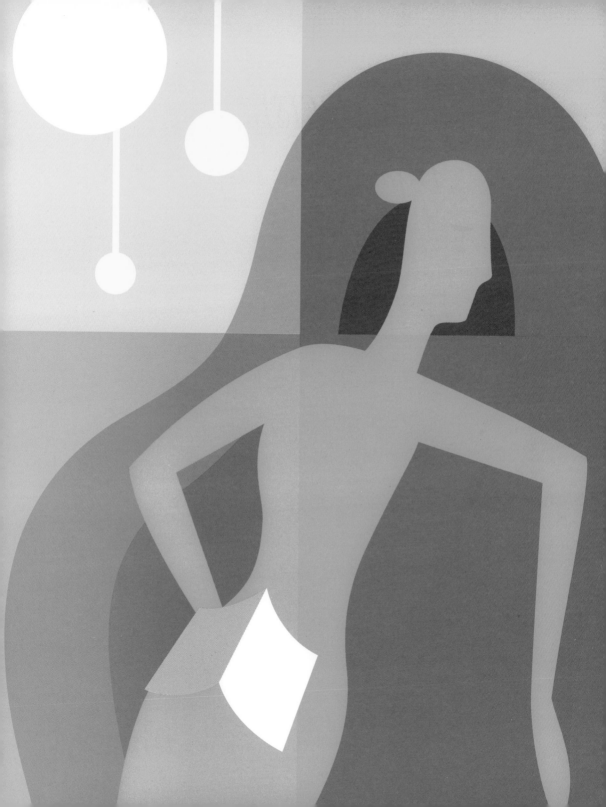

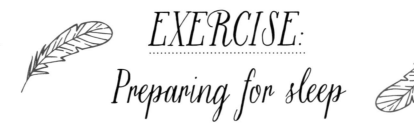

EXERCISE:
Preparing for sleep

Write down the ways in which you prepare for a good night's sleep:

_____

_____

_____

_____

_____

How could your routine be improved?

_____

_____

_____

_____

_____

QUICK GUIDE TO FALLING ASLEEP

Have you tried any of the following? Which ones work best for you?

- Clear your mind, meditate, chant and practise mindfulness.
- Count sheep.
- Do some relaxation exercises.
- Mentally go through the alphabet and think of two things that begin with each letter (animals, cities, movie stars, or whatever you like).
- Take a warm bath.
- Turn off electricals such as your TV, computer and phone at least an hour before your bedtime.
- Eat a banana or drink a mug of warm milk.
  Try a herbal supplement.
- Read a good book.
- Think positive thoughts.
- Buy some blackout curtains.
- Listen to soothing music or white noise, or use a noise-cancelling app.
- Wear an eye mask.
- Use ear plugs.
- Buy a good mattress.
- Keep the temperature of your bedroom cool.
- Wear cotton sleepwear.
- Try not to have an argument just before going to bed.
- Write down your thoughts in a journal.

Can you think of any other methods?

_____

_____

_____

_____

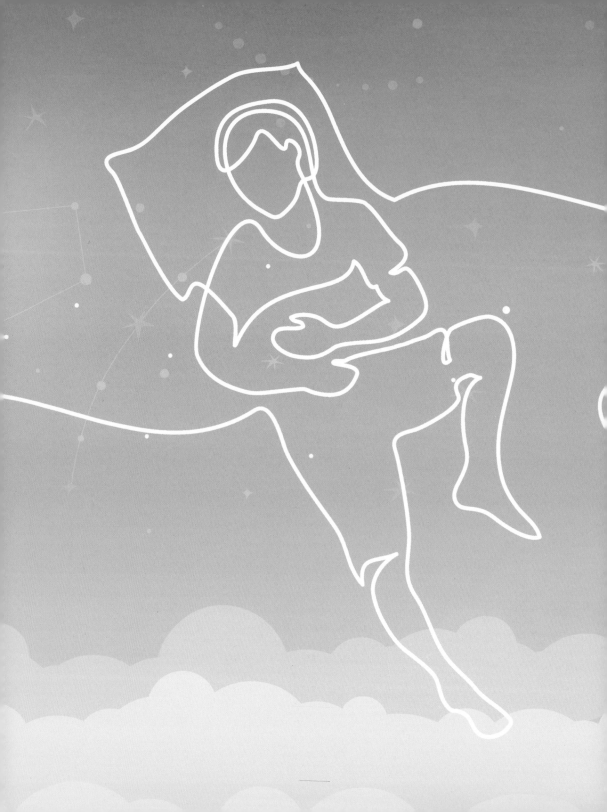

Part two
DREAM WELL

Having built up a healthy sleep program and started to enjoy regular sleep patterns, the second part of this journal explores the magical world of dreams. By keeping a dream diary and learning how to incubate and interpret your dreams, it's possible to tap into unconscious emotions and gain valuable insights into areas of your life that need attention, as well as behaviours or thought patterns that might be improved. Taking the time to record and understand your dreams is incredibly rewarding, offering the opportunity to access unconscious thoughts and comprehend hidden messages, and to delve into the deepest parts of your personality and find meaning.

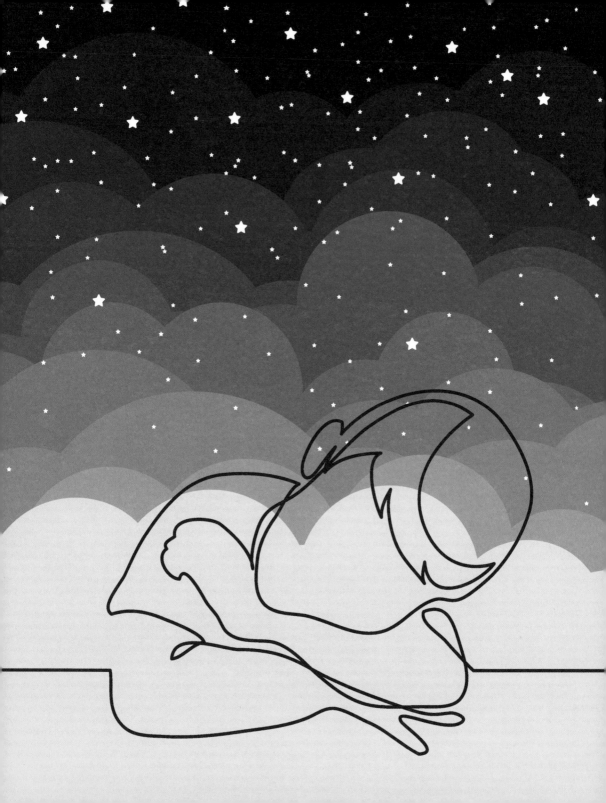

The process of dreaming

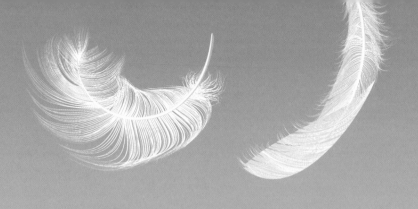

Why do we dream?

Dreams consist of the images and stories that our minds create while we're asleep. They can make us feel happy, sad, afraid or confused – and many other emotions besides. Sometimes dreams relate to everyday situations and people, but often they contain elements that seem perfectly rational at the time but on reflection are completely bizarre.

There are varying opinions as to why we dream. No one knows for sure, but scientific studies show that our health is compromised if we don't dream: people who are woken up just before entering the dream state are found to experience tension, depression, anxiety, problems concentrating, a lack of coordination and even weight gain, so dreams are important for our health and wellbeing.

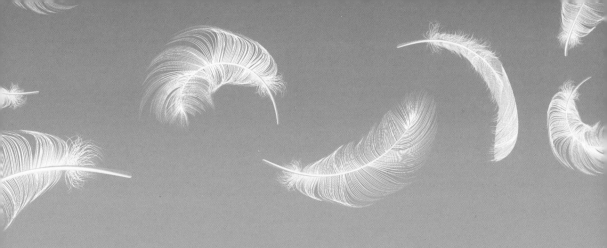

Here are a few theories about the reasons for dreaming – some cognitive, some psychological and some biological:

- Dreams help us to process our emotions and store the day's memories while simultaneously getting rid of any information we don't need.
- Dreams are an extension of our waking lives, continuing our conscious experience of the world while we're asleep. They may protect the mind from perceived danger, threats and challenges.
- They are a means by which we solve problems and achieve psychological and emotional balance. While dreaming, we are able to work through difficult, complex and unsettling thought processes. How many times have you gone to bed with a problem and woken up with the solution?
- Dreams are a part of normal brain activity – the brain's response to the biochemical changes and electrical impulses that occur when we're at rest.
- They are a window into our subconscious, revealing our unconscious desires, thoughts and motivations. Some people believe that dreams tap into a consciousness that unites our past, present and future.

What happens when we dream?

Dreaming usually occurs during the rapid eye movement (REM) stage of sleep, also known as Stage 4 sleep (see pages 14–15). During the course of a night, we may dream for up to two hours in total, but this is broken up four or five times by the sleep cycle. Throughout the night, each cycle progressively includes more REM sleep and less deep sleep.

Physiologically, several changes take place during REM sleep: our breathing and heart rate quicken, our blood pressure rises, we become less able to regulate our body temperature, we become immobilized (except for our eyes which move rapidly), and our brain activity increases to the same level as when we're awake – or sometimes even higher. Our vital signs indicate an aroused state, and our brain uses more oxygen than it does when we're awake.

Infants spend almost 50 per cent of their sleep time in REM sleep, while for adults this figure is around 20 per cent. This may be due to the huge amount of learning that takes place in infancy. Interestingly, we are not the only animals to dream; other mammals and also birds have REM sleep stages, which suggests that they dream too.

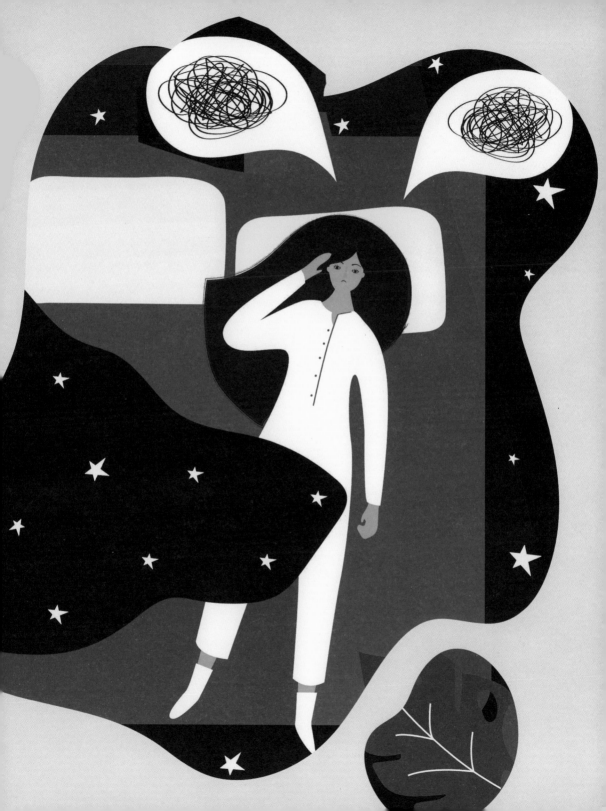

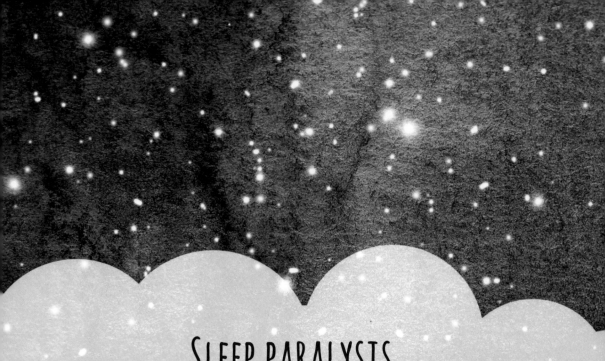

Sleep paralysis

· · · · · · · · · · · · · ☾ · · · · · · · · · ·

Immediately before, during and after periods of dreaming, our body becomes immobilized, and this paralysis lasts until we leave REM sleep. Normally we are unaware of it – and it's probably nature's way of ensuring that we don't act out our dreams and harm ourselves while dreaming – but occasionally we experience an inability to move or speak just as we're waking up or falling asleep, and it can be quite frightening.

During sleep paralysis we're essentially experiencing REM sleep while we're awake. We may feel pressure on our chest to the point where it's difficult to breathe, we may be unable to open our eyes, and we may have a strong sensation that there's someone or something malevolent in the room. An episode may last from a few seconds to several minutes, and might occur once or twice in a lifetime or up to several times a month.

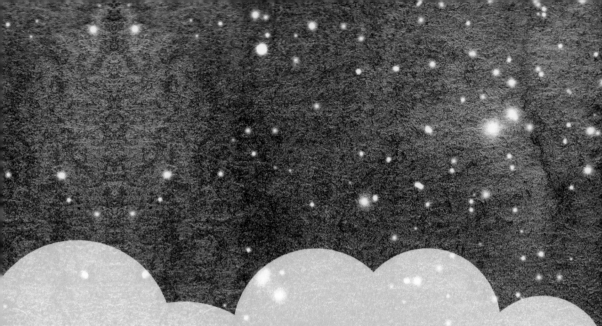

The causes of sleep paralysis include not getting enough sleep, sleeping at irregular times, jet lag, narcolepsy (falling asleep at inappropriate times), a family history of sleep paralysis, or sleeping on your back.

HOW TO DEAL WITH SLEEP PARALYSIS

- Keep to a set routine at bedtime – go to bed at roughly the same time each night and get up at the same time each morning.
- Adjust your sleeping environment so that it's quiet, dark, comfortable and a cool temperature.
- If you normally sleep on your back, try other positions.
- Exercise regularly, but not within four hours of bedtime.
- Avoid eating large meals and drinking caffeine or alcohol before bed.
- Make sure you're getting enough sleep; aim for seven to nine hours.
- If your sleep paralysis is severe or you feel anxious about it, see your doctor. You may be prescribed a low dose of antidepressant medication, which alters REM sleep.

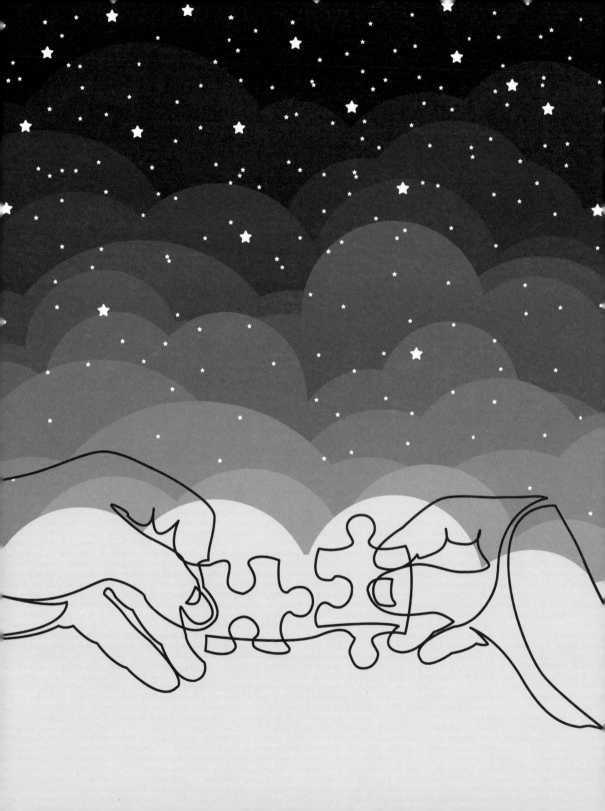

Managing your dreams

LUCID DREAMING

Normally when we're asleep, our brain seems to 'switch off' and we're not self-aware, but sometimes we can become conscious that we're dreaming – a state known as 'lucid dreaming'. It's been estimated that about 55 per cent of people have experienced this state at some point during their lifetime.

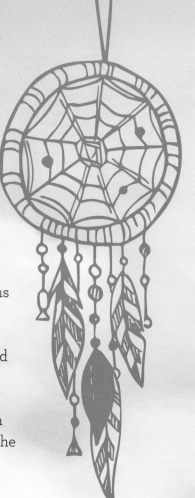

In terms of the sleep stages, lucid dreaming occurs between REM sleep and wakefulness, and is accompanied by increased activity in the parts of the brain that are usually suppressed during sleep.

Some people are actually able to train themselves to control their dreams and improve their lucidity while being half-asleep/half-awake. The American scientist Stephen LaBerge studied lucid dreaming in the 1970s and 80s and developed the 'mnemonic induction of lucid dreams' (MILD) technique, which enabled him and his subjects to enter the lucid state at will.

Waking early and then dozing for a while can often induce lucid dreaming, while some people achieve a better result by napping during the daytime. The best time for lucidity is probably during the final period of sleep, just before waking.

MNEMONIC INDUCTION OF LUCID DREAMS (MILD) TECHNIQUE

- While you're drifting off to sleep, think of a dream you've had recently.
- Notice something strange or bizarre in the dream, such as the ability to fly.
- Picture yourself returning to the dream, remembering that the bizarre element only occurs while you're dreaming.
- Repeat a mantra to yourself, such as: 'Tonight I will have a lucid dream.'

Asking for the dreams you want

· · · · · · · · · · · · · · · ☾ · · · · · · · · · · · · · ·

Once you've achieved lucidity while dreaming, it becomes possible to ask for the dreams you want – that is, to incubate your dreams. This can be done by 'planting a seed' in your mind in order to dream about a specific topic or solve a particular problem. A method known by the acronym CARDS (clarify, ask, repeat, dream, study) involves taking the following steps:

C Clarify the issue. An example might be: 'Promotion at work eludes me.'

A Ask the questions, 'who? what? where? when? why?'. For instance, you might ask:
- Who can best help in my search for promotion?
- What must I do to be in line for promotion?
- Where do the best opportunities lie for me?
- When will I be able to use my greater experience?
- Why is my expertise not being recognized?

R Repeat the questions over and over, to fix them in your subconscious mind. Blocks of three repetitions work well.

D Dream, then document your dream as soon as you wake up, noting down the main theme.

S Study the dream by looking at the imagery and thinking about any details, clues and hidden meanings, and see whether you can apply these to situations in your everyday life.

EXERCISE:
Target dream

Following the CARDS method on the previous page, write down what you would like to dream, then think about your target dream just before you are about to go to sleep.

_____

_____

_____

_____

_____

_____

_____

_____

_____

_____

_____

_____

The next morning, write down what you have dreamed.

_____

_____

_____

_____

_____

_____

_____

_____

What answers did your dream provide for each of your questions?

_____

_____

_____

_____

_____

_____

_____

_____

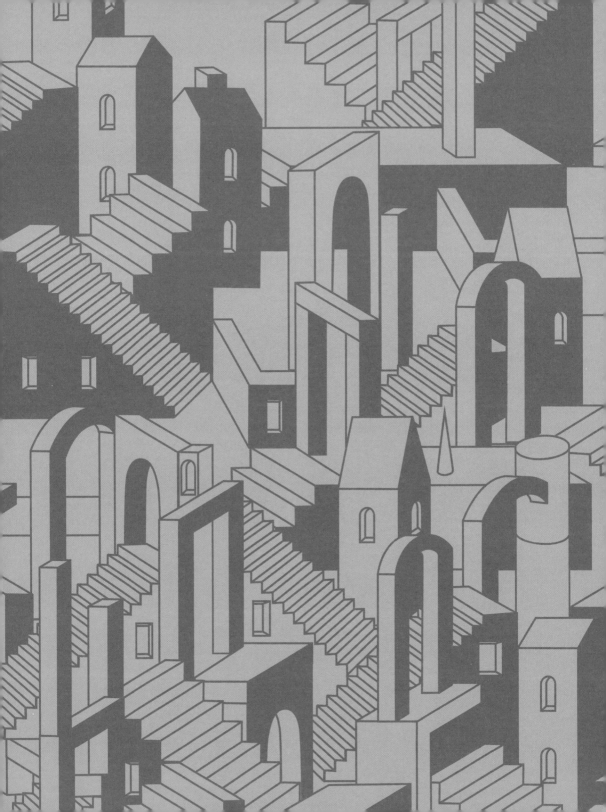

REALITY CHECK

Get into a day-time routine of checking to see if you are dreaming. This makes it more likely that you'll do this out of habit when you are actually dreaming. Then, when you ask yourself if you are dreaming and find that you are, you can explore the possibilities of your lucid dream state. You can do this in several ways:

- Look at your hands and feet. Are they the right sizes? If they seem larger or smaller than normal, you are probably dreaming.
- Look into a mirror to check if your reflection looks normal.
- Press against a solid object to see if your hand can go through it.
- Pinch your nose and check whether you can still breathe. If you can, you're dreaming.
- Look at a clock. The time may constantly change if you're dreaming, but if you're awake it will hardly change at all.
- Carry out an action that you know is impossible in real life, such as jumping an enormous distance or rolling up a hill. If you can perform the action, you are dreaming.
- Ask yourself repeatedly, 'Am I dreaming?'

These sorts of reality checks should ideally be done about 10 times a day. You could set an alarm every couple of hours to remind you to do your checks.

Dealing with nightmares

Nightmares are vivid, unpleasant dreams that evoke feelings of fear and distress. Common examples include being chased by someone, having your teeth fall out, sitting an exam and realizing you've forgotten to study, falling from a great height, discovering that you're naked in public, being attacked, or feeling like you're paralyzed or dying.

They usually pass quickly upon waking, but sometimes they can become a chronic problem that interfere with good-quality sleep. The good news is it's possible to 'change the story' using a method known by the acronym RISC (recognize, identify, stop, change):

- Recognize that you are having a bad dream, but that you don't need the negative feeling, whether it be fear, anger, embarrassment, guilt, or any other negative emotion.
- Identify exactly what is disturbing about the nightmare. What is making you feel bad?
- Stop the nightmare, either by waking up or becoming lucid (aware that you're dreaming). You can be in charge of your dreams, and you don't need to let a nightmare continue.
- Change the dream from negative feelings and actions to positive ones. Initially, you may only be able to do this when you're awake, but with practice you can learn to do it while remaining asleep.

Try to evoke images that trigger feelings of strength and power.

Bear in mind that nightmares can be caused by medications and anxiety conditions, or even something as simple as eating late at night – so if you do have an occasional bad dream, it's important to look into the possible biological or emotional reasons behind them.

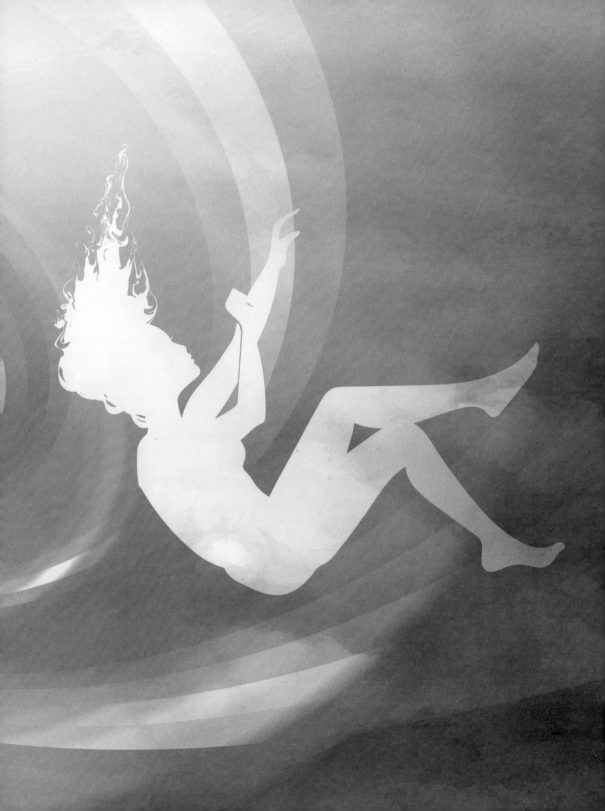

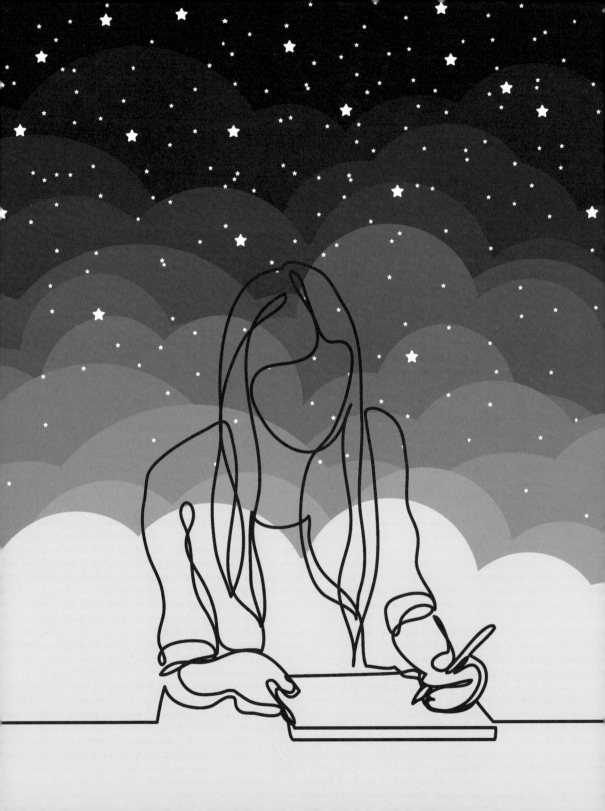

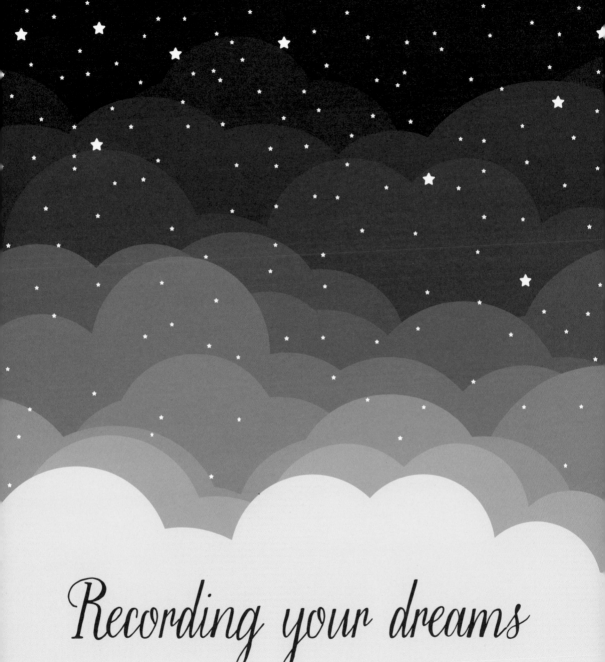

Recording your dreams

Significant dream

· · · · · · · · · · ☾ · · · · · · · · · · ·

Write out the details of a significant dream the morning after you have it. Keep this journal by your bedside so it is to hand when you wake up.

DATE:

....

OVERALL FEELING FROM THE DREAM:

....

_____

_____

_____

_____

_____

_____

_____

_____

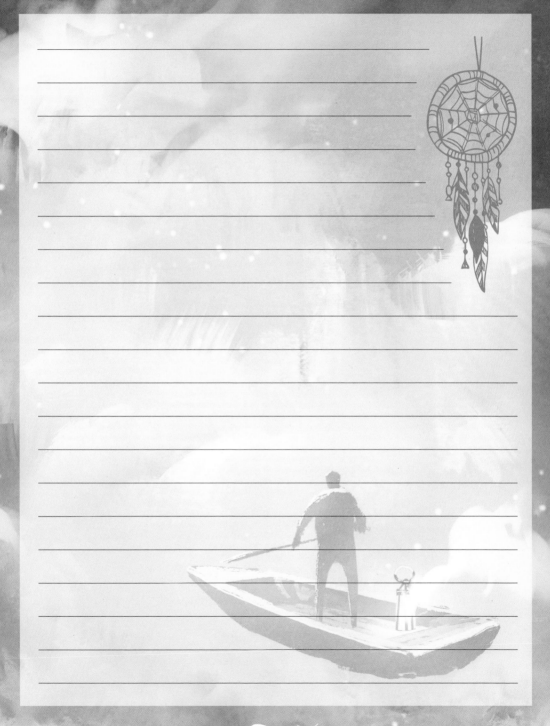

How to keep a dream journal

Once you start chronicling your dreams, you might be amazed to find that patterns occur, or that you tend to dream about certain subjects when you're in the midst of particular episodes in your life.

Dreams are notoriously quick to fade, so it's best to keep your journal and pen on your bedside table and make notes as soon as you wake up. Keep your descriptions succinct and clear, focusing on the events of the dream, your emotions, the people in the dream, and whether anything was strange within the dream. To help you remember it later, it's a good idea to give your dream a title.

Here's a simple template you could follow:

- Time and date.
- Dream title.
- What happened in the dream?
- What were your emotions and feelings?
- What people were in the dream? What were they doing?
- Write down anything odd or bizarre about the dream.

The more you practise recording your dreams, the easier it will become and the more details you will remember. Be relaxed about the process; don't stress if you can't remember every dream – you'll improve in time. It's an interesting fact that most people find that their dreams become much more vivid and colourful once they start writing them down.

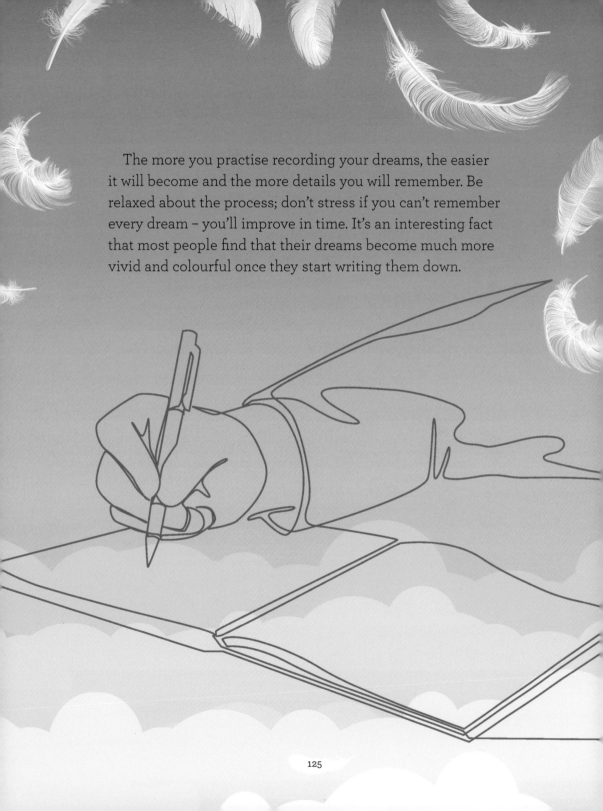

EXERCISE: My dream journal

Record your dreams for a week.

Monday

_____

_____

_____

_____

_____

_____

_____

_____

_____

_____

_____

_____

_____

Tuesday

_____

_____

_____

_____

_____

_____

_____

_____

_____

_____

_____

_____

_____

_____

_____

_____

_____

Wednesday

Thursday

Friday

Saturday

_____

_____

_____

_____

_____

_____

_____

_____

_____

_____

_____

_____

_____

_____

_____

_____

_____

_____

_____

_____

_____

_____

_____

Sunday

Make notes here about any recurring elements in the dreams you've had throughout the week, or anything you feel is significant.

_____

_____

_____

_____

_____

_____

_____

_____

_____

_____

_____

_____

_____

_____

_____

_____

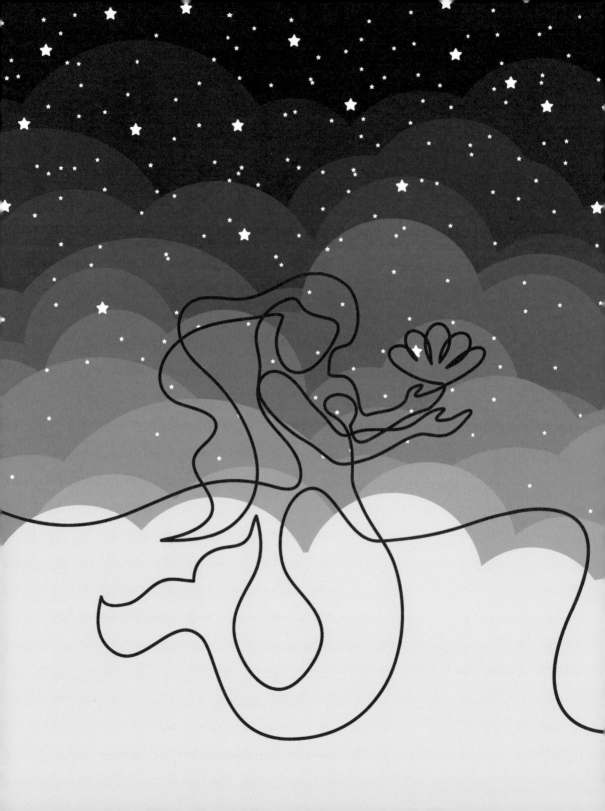

Analyzing your dreams

How to interpret your dreams

· · · · · · · · · · · · · ☾ · · · · · · · · · · ·

Everyone's dreams are unique to them, so there are no hard and fast rules about what particular dream scenarios mean. Generally, dreams help us to solve problems, come to terms with our emotions and seek out balance and harmony in life, and as such, the dreamer is the expert. In other words, *you are the best interpreter of your own dreams*.

An example of this is that the owl is considered a wise bird in many European cultures but is a term for a fool in India. This is because many European cultures have beliefs that originate in ancient Greek and Roman ideas. In this case, the owl is the symbol of Athena, the virgin goddess of wisdom. In India, however, the characteristic the owl has of sleeping during the day is believed to be representative of ignorance. Such cultural divergences mean that your personal background and beliefs will influence what a dream means to you.

Having said that, there are certain situations, symbols and themes that occur time and time again for many people in many different cultures. On the following pages, we identify the themes of the most common dreams and also give you some guidance on how to interpret them.

KEEP RECORDING

In the previous chapter (pages 124-5) we discovered how to keep a dream journal and did a week's worth of recording our dreams. Continue this practice in another notebook if you need more space, or on the following pages if relevant. The more you get into the habit of recording your dreams, the more you will remember them and be able to interpret them.

PEOPLE IN DREAMS

CELEBRITIES

Famous people are often in our minds, from musicians and movie stars to politicians or even historical figures, so it's not surprising that they feature in our dreams. When we meet a celebrity in a dream, it doesn't necessarily mean we're obsessed with that person; the celebrity is usually a symbol for an aspect of ourselves that may be lacking or that is important to us. For example, dreaming of a famous comedian may mean that we wish to be more confident or humorous.

EXERCISE: Have you ever met any famous people in your dreams?

_____

_____

What qualities do those celebrities possess?

_____

_____

_____

What do you think these dreams mean?

_____

_____

_____

MEETING OLD FRIENDS OR PEOPLE YOU KNOW

There are a few possibilities in interpreting dreams about family, friends and acquaintances. You may simply be thinking about someone and missing them, or you may feel the need to be admired by them. Alternatively, the characteristics of the familiar people in your dreams may be the qualities that you would like to have yourself.

EXERCISE: Which people in your social circle have you dreamt about?

_____

_____

_____

_____

_____

_____

What traits do they have that you would like to have?

_____

_____

_____

_____

_____

_____

_____

DANGERS IN DREAMS

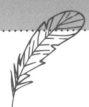

BEING CHASED

If you're being chased in a dream, you may be feeling threatened in your waking life and are running away from something that's causing you anxiety. The threat could be psychological, such as fear, anger or jealousy, or it could be an unresolved item on your 'to do' list, such as a piece of work you haven't finished. The message of the dream is that you need to pay attention and confront whatever issue is worrying you.

EXERCISE: If you've ever dreamt that you were being chased, who or what was chasing you?

_____

How did it make you feel?

_____

_____

_____

In what ways might your dream have been connected to events in your waking life?

_____

_____

_____

BEING TRAPPED OR BURIED ALIVE

The feeling of being confined means that you're anxious about your current situation and you feel restricted. This could apply to your job, friendship, romantic relationship or where you live. Being buried may refer to an untapped talent that you are yet to explore. The dream is telling you to think about changing your circumstances in some way or to try out a new activity.

EXERCISE: Describe a dream in which you felt confined or restricted.

_____

_____

_____

_____

_____

What was happening in your life at the time?

_____

_____

_____

_____

_____

Births and Deaths

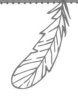

BABIES OR HAVING CHILDREN

Infants are associated with innocence, happiness and new beginnings, and a dream about a baby may herald an exciting future project or a new stage in your life. However, this is highly dependent on your feelings about babies and having children. If you are wanting a baby and are undergoing fertility treatment, it is only natural that your dreams will focus on this aspect of your life. If, however, babies represent being restricted or forced into responsibilities you are unwilling to take on, such a dream can be a sign that you are finding it difficult to say no. You may be launching a new business that you see as being 'your baby' and your dreams are literally showing you this.

EXERCISE: What do babies represent for you?

_____

_____

_____

_____

_____

_____

_____

_____

DYING

Dreaming about dying isn't necessarily fearful or related to death itself, but rather transformation and changes in your waking life. If you experience your own death in a dream, it often signals new beginnings and a fresh start – a chance to move on to something positive, such as marriage, a new job, a new home or recovery from a past relationship. Dying in a dream represents putting the past behind us, opening the door to a new stage of life.

EXERCISE: Have you ever dreamt that you or someone else has died? Describe your dream.

_____

_____

_____

How did you feel when you woke up? If you felt anxious, it could be that change makes you nervous rather than your dream being a prophesy about an actual death.

_____

_____

_____

_____

_____

FEARS TO ADDRESS

TEETH FALLING OUT

Dreaming that your teeth are falling out or crumbling is extremely common, and is thought to represent anxiety. On a physical level, it could relate to feelings of attractiveness – you might have worries about your physical appearance and the way other people perceive you, or you might be worried about getting older. It can also represent a fear of being embarrassed, making a fool of ourselves or being rejected in some way. Dreams like this typically occur when we feel unprepared for something and we're afraid of failing. They may originate from childhood, when we're anxious about losing our baby teeth.

EXERCISE: Have you ever dreamt about something strange in your appearance such as teeth or hair falling out? What happened in your dream?

_____

_____

Were you experiencing anxiety about any particular aspect of your life?

_____

_____

_____

_____

BEING LOST

The panicky feeling of being lost often arises in dreams when we're anxious, confused, vulnerable or insecure in our waking lives. The dream scenario might be a forest, a haunted house, a multi-storey car park, the dark or fog, and we repeatedly try to find our way home but can't. This type of dream often occurs when we don't know what to do next, when we're unable to escape a problem or don't know where to turn for help. It can also mean that we're too emotionally dependent on someone else and are afraid of losing them. The dream is telling us that we wish to reconnect with the things and people that make us happy.

EXERCISE: Who would you benefit from reconnecting with?

_____

_____

_____

_____

How might you go about making difficult decisions in your waking life? Could you make a list of pros and cons and decide that way?

_____

_____

_____

_____

_____

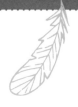

BEASTS AND BEASTLINESS

ANIMALS

Dreams about animals are often really dreams about aspects of our own personality. Different animals have their own specific characteristics, so a dream about a wild animal might represent the wilder part of our nature, while a dream about a pet might reflect our capacity for love and friendship. Animal dreams often reveal our hidden motives and emotions: a cat might symbolize creativity and independence; a dog loyalty and protection; a horse strength and power. Whichever animal we dream about, we're subconsciously thinking about our own behaviour in the waking world.

EXERCISE: Which animals have appeared in your dreams?

_____

_____

_____

What qualities do they possess?

_____

_____

_____

_____

_____

SNAKES AND SPIDERS

For obvious reasons, snakes are thought to symbolize either fear or sexual energy. If you dream of a snake, you may be afraid of a stressful situation or a confrontation with someone, or you may have unfulfilled desires or a need for intimacy. Snakes are also associated with transformation, so a snake dream could be a forewarning of a change coming in your life. Like snakes, spiders are also commonly feared, and dreaming of seeing a spider could represent the feeling of being trapped – perhaps in a relationship, a job or a financial situation.

EXERCISE: Whether you fear or like snakes and spiders will affect your interpretation of dreams about them. How do you feel about snakes and spiders in your waking life?

_____

_____

Describe a dream you've had about creepie-crawlies.

_____

_____

_____

Was it a dream or a nightmare? How did it make you feel?

_____

_____

_____

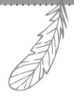

Sensations in dreams

FLYING

Flying is thought to reflect the amount of control you have in your everyday life. You might dream that you're flying when you feel somewhat out of control in your waking life. A dream in which you can fly is sending you a message of hope and freedom – that nothing is impossible, and you can do anything you want to in order to reach your goals. Thus, flying dreams can provide motivation when you need it.

EXERCISE: What would you like to feel motivated to do?

_____

_____

_____

_____

_____

Which physical sensations in dreams have made you feel free and happy?

_____

_____

_____

_____

_____

FALLING

Virtually everyone has dreamt of falling at one time or another. It is thought that falling is an indication of insecurities, worries and feelings of being overwhelmed by events in our waking life. It signals that we're not in control of a particular situation and that we feel helpless. A dream of falling tells us that we need to be open to changes and take responsibility for our actions.

EXERCISE: Describe a dream in which you were falling.

_____

_____

How did the fall begin – did you lose your balance or were you pushed?

_____

How did you land, or did you keep falling indefinitely?

_____

How did you feel while you were falling?

_____

In what ways do you think your answers to these questions might affect how you'd interpret your dream?

_____

_____

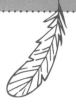

Loss of Control

BEING UNABLE TO MOVE

Being frozen to the spot, paralyzed or stuck in mud or concrete is a very common dream. Paralysis is part of the normal sleep process as we enter REM sleep (see pages 106–7), but dreaming about being unable to move is usually about control. Not being able to move your legs or trying to run but not getting anywhere both suggest that you're not in control of your life. You may have goals that you're not reaching, you may feel stuck in your career or pattern of behaviour, you may be experiencing setbacks, or you may be procrastinating. If so, it's probably time to reconsider what you want in life, and how you might get closer to making this a reality.

EXERCISE: Make some notes about any dreams in which you felt stuck – were you experiencing a stalling in your life at that time?

_____

_____

_____

Is there an area of your life in which you'd like to move forward? Incubate a dream to give you guidance (pages 112-13).

_____

_____

_____

_____

BEING IN A RUNAWAY CAR

Driving a car in a dream denotes life's journey and the ability to navigate from one stage to another, so dreaming that the vehicle is out of control suggests that you're not happy with the way things are going and you're veering off track. You may be spending too much time focusing on other people's problems or trying to make other people happy, when you really should be paying attention to your own life and taking control of your own destiny. Similarly, if you dream that your car's brakes aren't working, it suggests a lack of control – perhaps your workload has got out of hand or you're worried about a relationship. Your dream is reminding you that these issues need addressing.

EXERCISE: What sort of car dreams have you had?

_____

_____

Did you ever discover that you couldn't reach the brake pedal, or that there was something wrong with the car?

_____

How did you feel?

_____

Were you ever the passenger rather than the driver? What do you think this might mean?

_____

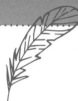

Embarrassing situations

BEING UNPREPARED

The feeling of being unprepared in a dream can take many forms. You might dream that you've just sat down in an exam room and realized that you forgot to study beforehand, or that you've walked on stage to perform a play and you've forgotten your lines. Sir Laurence Olivier admitted to a version of this, in which he would hear his cue and open the door to the set, but discover that the door led to another door, then another door, and another, and he would never make it to the stage. These are all anxiety dreams that share the theme of being 'put to the test' in some way. They may represent the fear of taking the next step in your life, or be reminders that you need to prepare for important challenges to come.

EXERCISE: Virtually all actors have experienced the dream in which they make their stage entrance and then go completely blank. Have you ever felt lost for words or unable to complete a task in a dream? How did you feel when you woke up?

_____

_____

Did you take any action in your waking life as a result (extra studying if you found yourself unable to take an exam in your dream)?

_____

_____

BEING NAKED IN PUBLIC

This is an acutely embarrassing and shocking situation to find yourself in – the idea that you're in public and suddenly realize that you're not wearing any clothes. A dream like this often crops up when we're promoted or start a new job, since this is a time when we feel vulnerable and 'on show'. If you're worried about your appearance or what people think of you, the dream could be telling you that you're trying to be something you're not. Look deeply into yourself to find out whether you need to change, or whether you're fine as you are.

EXERCISE: List some of the ways in which you could reduce your anxiety about how others perceive you.

_____

_____

_____

_____

_____

_____

_____

_____

_____

EXERCISE:

My most memorable dreams

Use the remaining pages in this journal to record your most vivid dreams. For each one, make a note about what type of dream it is – for example, it might be a recurring dream (perhaps from childhood), an anxiety dream or a premonition of the future.

Then write a short paragraph describing what the dream means to you. It's worth repeating here: *you are the best interpreter of your own dreams.*

INDEX